The Sexual Secrets

In this book you and your partner will learn

How women can have multiple orgasms every time

and overcome difficulties having orgasms

How men can have multiple orgasms without losing their erection

and overcome problems with erection and premature ejaculation

How both of you can have longer, more intense whole-body orgasms

and have more desire, energy, and creativity

How to harmonize male and female desire and satisfy each other fully

and the arts of genital massage, oral sex, and thrusting

How sex can heal you and keep you young

and sexual positions for harmonizing and healing

How to connect love and lust

and cultivate love for each other

How to experience Soul-Mating and Soul Orgasms

and the importance of sexuality for your spiritual relationship

How to maintain the sexual charge in your relationship

and cultivate passion and pleasure over a lifetime of lovemaking

THE MULTI-ORGASMIC COUPLE

THE

Sexual Secrets

MULTI-

Every Couple

ORGASMIC

Should Know

COUPLE

**Mantak Chia,
Maneewan Chia
Douglas Abrams,
and Rachel Carlton Abrams, M.D.**

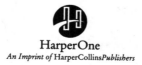

HarperOne
An Imprint of HarperCollins*Publishers*

HarperOne

HarperCollins books may be purchased for educational, business, or sales promotional use. For information please e-mail the Special Markets Department at SPsales@harpercollins.com.

HarperCollins Web site: http://www.harpercollins.com

HarperCollins®, 📖®, and HarperOne™ are trademarks of HarperCollins Publishers.

Illustrations by John Raynes

FIRST HARPERCOLLINS PAPERBACK EDITION PUBLISHED IN 2002

Library of Congress Cataloging-in-Publication Data
Chia, Mantak.
   The multi-orgasmic couple : sexual secrets every couple
should know / Mantak Chia . . . [et al.].
   p. cm.
   Includes biographical references.
ISBN 978–0–06–251614–5
   1. Sex instruction. 2. Sex in marriage. 3. Sexual excitement. I. Title.
HQ31.C534   2001
613.9'6—dc21   00–039617

23 24 25 26 27 LBC 47 46 45 44 43

CONTENTS

CHAPTER EIGHT
Making Love for a Lifetime   177

WARNING: *These are powerful practices.* The techniques given in this book can profoundly improve your health as well as your sexuality. However, we do not give any diagnoses or suggestions for medication. If you have a medical condition, a medical doctor should be consulted. People who have high blood pressure, heart disease, or a generally weak condition should proceed slowly in the practice. If you have questions about or difficulty with the practice, you should contact a Universal Tao instructor in your area (see Resources: Universal Tao Books and Instructors).

Practice makes pleasure. Because this book is based on a three-thousand-year tradition of actual sexual experience, the authors are well aware of the effort that is involved—pleasurable as it may be—in changing your sex life. Learning sexual secrets is one thing, but using them is quite another. The techniques in this book have been tested and refined by countless lovers over thousands of years in the laboratory of real life. We have tried to present them in as clear and simple a way as possible, but the only way to benefit from them is to really use them.

It may help to know a little about the authors to better understand the book and the many benefits of multi-orgasmic lovemaking. Let us begin by explaining how we came to write this book with Mantak and Maneewan Chia, since we never set out to write a sex book.

We stumbled across Taoist sexuality while Rachel was entering medical school and Doug was studying and working ten-hour days. We were amazed not only at the far more pleasurable and profound lovemaking we experienced but also at the increased energy we had for our work and our lives as a whole.

Taoist sexuality, also called the "Arts of the Bedchamber," is a three-thousand-year-old tradition that has long known about male multiple orgasms and many other secrets of sexual satisfaction. It was developed to help couples experience more pleasurable and more healing lovemaking. With all the shame and misinformation that most of us grow up with about our sexuality, the Taoist Arts of the Bedchamber were a revelation.

We shared the existing books on Taoist sexuality with our friends, who said the practice sounded wonderful but they didn't know how or where to begin. Unfortunately, there was no simple step-by-step book that showed ordinary men and women like us how to become multi-orgasmic and how to experience the physically healing, emotionally intimate, and spiritually profound aspects of lovemaking. Finally, after many requests from friends, we agreed to try and write such a book.

After extensive reading and research, it was clear that Mantak and Maneewan Chia were the most authentic and practical teachers of this tradition. Mantak Chia had studied for many years with Taoist masters, learning the sexual wisdom that he distilled into a unique system he called "Healing Love." Its benefits are greater healing and love as well as greater pleasuring and passion. He has taught thousands of people around the world, has trained hundreds of teachers, and is respected as the world's leading teacher of Taoist sexuality, as well as powerful Taoist practices such as tai chi, chi kung, and others.

The Taoists masters, we quickly learned, were themselves physicians who studied sexual response with precision and insight. We were interested in

> Taoist sexuality, also called the "Arts of the Bedchamber," is a three-thousand-year-old tradition that has long known about male multiple orgasms and many other secrets of sexual satisfaction.

concrete benefits that people could experience in their own bedroom, as were they. We wanted to join the Taoist understanding and techniques, which have been refined over several thousand years, with the latest in scientific research.

We decided to write a book primarily for men, which was eventually called *The Multi-Orgasmic Man*, because much of the power of Healing Love depends on the man's ability to cultivate his sexuality and ideally to become multi-orgasmic. The book struck a chord and has been read by hundreds of thousands of readers around the world in more than ten languages.

While we were discussing the first book with readers around the country, we were continually asked when we would write a book for couples that would help women as well as men to incorporate Healing Love into their lives. Finally, several years and countless drafts later, we offer *The Multi-Orgasmic Couple*. We hope we have done justice to this rich tradition, presenting modern readers with the sexual wisdom we so desperately need in these days of carnal confusion.

This book has benefited from the expertise, wisdom, and skill of many people, who we would like to thank and acknowledge: the Universal Tao instructors who teach these practices around the world and who contributed to this book, including Michael Winn, Marcia Kerwit, and B. J. Santerre; the Eastern and Western sexologists whose research made this book possible, including Felice Dunas, Beverly Whipple, and Theresa Crenshaw; the extraordinary publishing team at HarperSanFrancisco, including John Loudon, Terri Leonard, Lisa Zuniga, Priscilla Stuckey, Karen Stough, Joseph Rutt, Joan Olson, Steve Kennedy, Kris Ashley, Calla Devlin, Margery Buchanan, Laura Beers, Jim Warner, Kathi Goldmark, Sam Barry, and Steve Hanselman; the readers, friends, and advisors who improved the manuscript, including Megory Anderson and Heather Kuiper; and our agent, Heide Lange, who has all three qualities—expertise, wisdom, and skill—in equal and extraordinary measure.

Finally, we would like to thank the readers, both men and women, of *The Multi-Orgasmic Man*, who have told us how the Arts of the Bedchamber have transformed their sexuality. We hope you and your partner (or future partner) find the joy and satisfaction that we have in this extremely powerful and profound practice of Healing Love.

Douglas Carlton Abrams
Rachel Carlton Abrams
Santa Cruz, California
April 17, 2000

Shocking as it is for most people to hear, both women *and men* can have multiple orgasms. In this book, both you and your partner will learn how to experience multiple whole-body orgasms. However, this is just the beginning of the sexual knowledge that we present. When you and your partner are both multi-orgasmic, you will each experience far greater individual pleasure. You will also be able to harmonize your sexual needs and to reach ever more fulfilling levels of intimacy and ecstasy together.

Multiple Orgasms for *All* Men

Few people know that men can have multiple orgasms. While this fact has been known for several thousand years in the East and has been confirmed in the West by Alfred Kinsey and other sex researchers since the 1940s,[1] it still remains a surprise to most men and women.

In our earlier book, *The Multi-Orgasmic Man*, we reviewed the most recent scientific evidence and presented ancient techniques for helping men become multi-orgasmic. We tried to give men a manual for a healthier and more satisfying experience of male sexuality. In this new book, we have tried to give couples a guidebook, or what the Taoists called "a pillow book," to deepen both partners' ability to experience pleasure, health, and intimacy.

Male multiple orgasms have been confirmed by Alfred Kinsey and other sex researchers since the 1940s.

Multiple Orgasms for *All* Women

While the fact that women can have multiple orgasms is well known, more than 50 percent of women have never had multiple orgasms or are not regularly multiply orgasmic. In this book, we will show all women how they can become consistently multi-orgasmic, and for those who are already multi-orgasmic we will show them how to expand and intensify their orgasms.

Harmonizing Sexual Desire

Lovemaking in which both partners are multi-orgasmic allows couples to reach many peaks of orgasmic pleasure together. Equally important, it allows

Multi-orgasmic lovemaking allows men and women to harmonize their often different sexual rhythms and desires.

men and women to harmonize their often different sexual rhythms and desires so that they can have a deeply satisfying and profoundly intimate love life.

But sensual pleasure, as exquisite and enjoyable as it can be, is only the beginning.

Physical Health, Emotional Intimacy, and Spiritual Growth

This book draws on thousands of years of sexual knowledge to show couples how sexual energy can be used to cultivate all other aspects of their relationship, including their physical health, emotional intimacy, and even spiritual growth. In the modern world, we have torn ourselves apart: we have separated our genitals from the rest of our body and our body from our spirit. In this book we show couples how to put the pieces together again for a level of health, intimacy, and spiritual union that many may never have known was possible.

The Loss of Sexual Wisdom

We live in a time of great sexual freedom but also great sexual confusion.

In the modern world, we have lost most of our sexual wisdom. We live in a time of great sexual freedom but also great sexual confusion. Sexuality is everywhere used to titillate us, but there remains an enormous amount of shame. Many readers may feel embarrassed about simply picking up a book on sexuality (*multiple orgasms*, no less!) in the bookstore. This is understandable since most of our churches, synagogues, mosques, and temples view sex through a narrow lens of fear and moralism. Most of us are left feeling profoundly anxious if not downright ashamed of our sexual needs and desires.

Even people with "healthy" attitudes toward sex still find it difficult to talk with their partner about what they want sexually. We may have little problem telling our partner where to rub our shoulders, but most of us are much more reticent to tell our partner where to rub our "privates." A major part of overcoming the shame that restricts our sexuality is learning that it is natural and discovering a more holistic and healthier view of human sexuality.

Discovering Sexual Wisdom

In this book, we present the sexual wisdom of the Taoist (pronounced DOW-*ist*) tradition. Originally, the Taoists were a group of seekers in ancient China (around 500 B.C.E.) who were devoted to understanding health and spirituality. In this book, we will call the Taoist sexual tradition "Healing Love" since lovemaking was seen as a powerful way to heal ourselves and each other. It was also called "Sexual Kung Fu." *Kung Fu* simply means "practice," so *Sexual Kung Fu* simply means "sexual practice." (Rest assured, you will *not* be breaking any bricks with your forehead or karate-chopping each other in bed.)

Sex Is About Health

The Taoists were doctors and were concerned with the body's overall well-being as much as with its sexual pleasure. For the Taoist then and now, sex is about health, not morality.

For the Taoists, sex is about health, not morality.

The Taoists deeply investigated the healing power of lovemaking. In addition to giving their patients pills, Taoist doctors would often prescribe making love in various positions to help cure different illnesses.

Taoist sexuality—or, as we will call it in this book, Healing Love—began as an important branch of Chinese medicine, and an active sex life was understood to be an essential part of health and longevity. In studies of older adults, modern medicine has recently confirmed that sex is in fact vital for our long-term health.

Among the early Taoists, sex was a serious science to be studied and understood like any other branch of medicine. In this way, the Taoists were like proto-sexologists, early Masters and Johnsons, you might say. Just as we study nutrition to prepare healthy food and study cooking to prepare delicious food, one was expected to study sexuality to make it both healthful and more enjoyable.

Sexual Harmony and Love for a Lifetime

The Taoists saw sexual harmony as essential for marital satisfaction. Indeed, this was one of the prime motivations in the development of the bedroom arts. They knew, like any modern-day couples' therapist, if there are problems in the bedroom the whole relationship suffers. Sexual harmony, however, is not always easy to achieve. Partners often have very different sexual needs. While

not all women or all men are identical, it was understood that women's sexual
arousal and sexual response often differ dramatically from men's.

The Taoists referred to these differences as the result of male and female
sexual energy (which they called *yang* and *yin*). We will explain to couples
how these energies influence our sexuality and how to use this understanding to satisfy both partners' needs.

It is worth mentioning that while the Taoists were primarily concerned
with harmonizing male and female sexuality, the practices are equally valuable for gay and lesbian couples. For the Taoists, all people have masculine
(yang) and feminine (yin) energy, and they knew it is essential for couples—
straight, gay, or lesbian—to harmonize the differences that exist between the
partners. In addition, the practices for pleasure, healing, emotional intimacy,
and spiritual relationship are equally powerful and important for gay and lesbian couples.

A New Sexual Evolution

While many of the Taoist practices for sexual fulfillment and physical
health are now over two thousand years old, they remain extremely effective
today. Over the past twenty years, since these long-secret Arts of the Bedchamber have started to be introduced to modern couples, there has been a
quiet but profound sexual evolution in bedrooms and in relationships around
the world. We hope the sexual arts and sexual science that we present in this
book will help your relationship as they have helped the thousands of others
who have practiced them.

Before you and your partner can explore the heights of Healing Love, it is
important for each partner to cultivate his or her own sexual potential. In
Part 1, "Solo: Multiplying and Expanding Your Orgasms," we first discuss how
both men and women can become multi-orgasmic. Then, in chapter 3, we discuss how couples can expand their sexual energy to experience whole-body
orgasms. The ability to circulate energy in your body will be important for the
practices introduced in Part 2, "Duo: Sharing Passion, Healing, and Intimacy
with Your Partner."

Solo:

Multiplying and

Expanding Your

Orgasms

CHAPTER 1

Fireworks: Multiple Orgasms for Men

In this chapter, you will discover:

- How to Separate Orgasm from Ejaculation
- How to Develop Sexual Strength and Sexual Sensitivity to Orgasm Without Ejaculating
- How to Become Multi-Orgasmic

Any man can become multi-orgasmic. It just takes a basic understanding of male sexuality and some simple techniques.* Multiple orgasms are extremely pleasurable and can expand a man's orgasmic experience. They also open a new sexual world to a man and his partner. For most men, their sexuality remains focused on the ultimately disappointing goal of ejaculating rather than on the orgasmic process of lovemaking. When a man becomes multi-orgasmic he is not only able to greatly satisfy himself, he is also much more able to fully satisfy his partner. Becoming multi-orgasmic is one of the greatest gifts a man can give his partner. It will help women to help their partners if they also read this chapter, so they too can understand this still little known ability that their partners are developing.

When a man becomes multi-orgasmic he is not only able to greatly satisfy himself, he is also much more able to fully satisfy his partner.

Orgasm and Ejaculation

Orgasm and ejaculation are different.

To become a multi-orgasmic man, you need to understand some basic facts about your anatomy. The most important fact is that orgasm and ejaculation are different. This is so startling to most men (and women) that we need to explain exactly how they are different. Let us begin by defining orgasm and ejaculation. Physiologically, an orgasm is the contraction and pulsation that most men feel in their penis, prostate, and pelvic area. It is accompanied by an increased heart rate, breathing rate, and blood pressure and results in a sudden release of tension.[1]

Obviously, orgasm is much more than these rather mechanical physiological changes. It is the peak experience of sex for most people, and it is one of the most intense and pleasurable parts of being human. If you have ever had an orgasm, and almost all men have, you know exactly what we are describing.

Ejaculation, however, is simply a reflex that occurs at the base of the spine and results in the ejection of semen. It is, in short, simply an involuntary muscle spasm.

Granted, it is a pleasurable muscle spasm, but it is a muscle spasm nonetheless. Since so many men have learned to connect all the pleasure of orgasm with ejaculation, it is important to understand that most of the lightning and thunder that you associate with ejaculation is really what occurs with orgasm—with or without ejaculation.

---

*In this chapter, we briefly summarize the information presented in our first book. For a longer and more detailed discussion of male multiple orgasms, please see the first three chapters of *The Multi-Orgasmic Man.*

In a moment we will review the scientific evidence that shows that men can have multiple orgasms, but it may be easier to begin with your own experience. In fact, you may have experienced multiple orgasms at some time in your life. Many men experience them before they enter adolescence and begin to ejaculate.

As you may remember, boys only start to produce sperm (and therefore the ability to ejaculate) once they enter adolescence, usually around the age of thirteen. However, most boys masturbate before they reach this age. During this time, they experience orgasm without ejaculating.

Many boys continue to masturbate after one orgasm, and since they do not ejaculate they maintain their erection. Alfred Kinsey, the pioneering sex researcher, in his famous book *Sexual Behavior in the Human Male* reported that half of all preadolescent boys (around twelve or younger) were able to experience two orgasms in a row, and almost a third were able to experience five or more one after the other. He concluded that "climax is clearly possible without ejaculation."[2]

Multiple orgasms, however, are not simply child's play or one of the lost pleasures of youth. Kinsey studied older men as well and concluded, "Orgasm may occur without the emission of semen. . . . These males experience real orgasm which they have no difficulty in recognizing, even if it is without ejaculation."[3] Dr. Herant Katchadourian, professor of human sexuality at Stanford University and the author of the standard textbook *Fundamentals of Human Sexuality*, explains, "Some men are able to inhibit the emission of semen [avoid ejaculating] while they experience the orgasmic contractions: in other words they have non-ejaculatory orgasms. Such orgasms do not seem to be followed by a refractory period [loss of erection], thereby allowing these men to have consecutive or multiple orgasms like women."[4]

There have long been anecdotal studies of men who claim to have multiple orgasms, but the first laboratory study of male multiple orgasms was conducted by sex researchers William Hartman and Marilyn Fithian. They tested thirty-three multi-orgasmic men—men who could have two or more orgasms without losing their erection.

While the men had sex with their partners, Hartman and Fithian monitored their heart rate, which rises from around 70 beats per minute during rest to 120 beats per minute during orgasm (see chart on p. 6). They also measured their pelvic contractions (which could be monitored through the involuntary squeezing of the anus that accompanies orgasm). They found that the arousal charts for multi-orgasmic men were exactly the same as for multi-orgasmic women.

Half of all preadolescent boys were able to experience two orgasms in a row, and almost a third were able to experience five or more one after the other.

Arousal chart for multi-orgasmic man

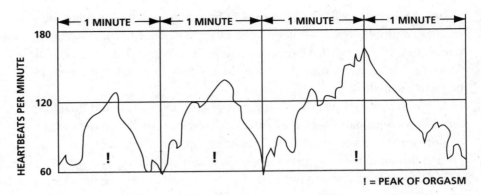

In one study, the average number of orgasms a multi-orgasmic man had was four. Some had the minimum of two, and one had sixteen.

In Hartman and Fithian's study, the average number of orgasms a multi-orgasmic man had was four. Some had the minimum of two, and one had sixteen. In another study, by sex researchers Marion Dunn and Jan Trost, most men reported having between two and nine orgasms before losing their erection.[5]

In their famous book, *The G-Spot and Other Recent Discoveries About Human Sexuality*, Alice Ladas, Beverly Whipple, and John Perry argued that male and female sexuality were much more similar than we tend to think. In addition to their discovery of the G spot, they also reported that men could have multiple orgasms like women. We tend to think that male sexuality is simple and identical from one man to the next, while female sexuality is complex and differs dramatically from one woman to the next. The truth is that ejaculation is simple, as are all bodily reflexes (think of hitting your funny bone), but orgasm, which involves our most sophisticated sexual organ, the brain, is quite complex and variable depending on the person, the sexual experience, and even the individual orgasm.

So, if men can have multiple orgasms like women and half of all boys experience multiple orgasms before adolescence, what happens that makes them lose this ability?

Apparently, most men lose the ability to have multiple orgasms when they start ejaculating in adolescence. Orgasm and ejaculation take place within seconds of each other and for most men become one and the same. In the next section, you will learn (or possibly relearn) how to separate the two once again. This will allow you to experience the crescendo of orgasm many times before or even without the crash of ejaculation.

Understanding Your Orgasm

Now that you understand the difference between orgasm and ejaculation, it is important to understand the nature of male orgasms and how multiple (non-ejaculatory) orgasms differ from the old-fashioned (ejaculatory) ones.

Multiple orgasms begin like any others: you start by getting aroused until you feel close to the point of ejaculating. As you learn in the following sections to increase your awareness of your arousal, you will be able to stop the stimulation just before the "point of no return," after which you would ejaculate. Just before this point, you will experience a series of contractions in your genitals lasting three to five seconds. These pleasurable pelvic orgasms at first may feel like a fluttering or a rather mild release of pressure. These are called "contractile-phase" orgasms, and in time as you learn to play with the edge they can be just as intense as the ejaculatory orgasms you are accustomed to. Don't get discouraged if they are rather tame at first. Once you are able to identify and separate these orgasmic contractions from ejaculation, you will be able to multiply and intensify them.

This contractile-phase orgasm is the moment of truth: instead of continuing on to ejaculation, you will stop or decrease your stimulation long enough to regain control of your arousal rate. You can also squeeze your PC muscle, which we will describe below, which will help you maintain some control if you feel like you are about to ejaculate.

With multiple orgasms, instead of cresting over into ejaculation, you will then decrease your arousal slightly and prepare for another orgasm. With multiple orgasms, your arousal is like a wave that instead of cresting is swept up by a larger wave that takes it even higher. Some multi-orgasmic men describe falling back into their orgasm rather than falling forward into ejaculation. These are simply metaphors that may help you as you discover your own orgasmic process.

It is important to remember not to strive too hard to experience these contractile-phase orgasms. Most men find they must stop themselves just before ejaculating and *relax* into orgasm. It is not easy for many men to switch their focus from the goal of getting off, but multiple orgasms allow you to experience an orgasmic process that is far more satisfying for you and your partner.

In the following section, we will show you how to strengthen your PC muscle and how to develop your sexual sensitivity so you can multiply and intensify your own unique orgasmic potential.

Multiplying Your Orgasm

In this book we discuss two ways to intensify your sexual pleasure. The first is by *multiplying* your orgasms (having two, three, four, or more without losing your erection), and the second is by *expanding* your orgasm throughout your body, which we will discuss in chapter 3. In learning to multiply your orgasms, you need to develop both your *sexual strength* and your *sexual sensitivity*. Let's look at sexual strength first.

DEVELOPING YOUR SEXUAL STRENGTH

Many men spend years strengthening their biceps and quads and other muscles to look strong, but there is one unseen muscle that will help them far more in bed than any other. This "sex muscle" is actually the pubococcygeus, or PC, muscle. This group of muscles runs from your pubic bone ("pubo") in the front of your body to the tailbone, or coccyx ("coccygeus"), in the back (see illustration on p. 9).

These muscles are essential for your sexual health. Two or three inches of your penis are rooted in this PC muscle, and strengthening this muscle leads to stronger erections, stronger orgasms, and better ejaculatory control. This last benefit is why the PC muscle is essential to becoming multi-orgasmic. In short, you will use the PC muscle to literally put on the brakes when you feel that you are getting close to ejaculating.

The easiest place to feel your PC muscle is behind your testicles and in front of your anus at your perineum. You are already well acquainted with your PC muscle, although you may not know its name. The PC muscle is the same muscle that you use to stop yourself from urinating or to push out the last few drops of urine.

Most important for multiple orgasms, the PC muscle is also what causes the rhythmic contractions in your pelvis and anus during orgasm. These pelvic contractions, the Taoists discovered, involved a man's prostate gland. By learning to contract your PC muscle around your prostate, you can learn to stop yourself from ejaculating and can deepen your orgasmic contractions. When you contract on the prostate, you feel a shaking or chill through your body. In the next section you are going to learn a simple exercise that will allow you to stop the stream of urine and strengthen your PC muscle.

> **You will use your PC muscle to literally put on the brakes when you feel that you are getting too close to ejaculating.**

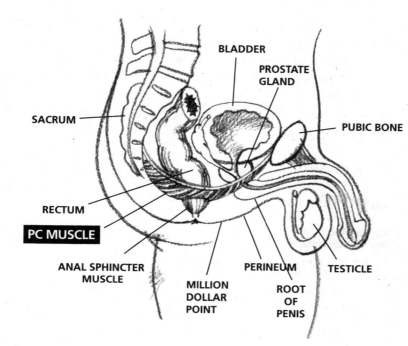

Man's Sexual Anatomy—the PC *muscle, which is important for becoming multi-orgasmic, extends from the pubic bone to the tailbone.*

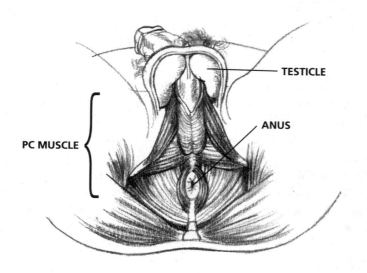

Another view of the PC *muscle (actually a group of muscles)*

STOPPING THE STREAM

The simplest way to find and strengthen your PC muscle is to squeeze these muscles in your pelvis the next time you are going to the bathroom. You can practice this while standing up or sitting down. If you have a relatively strong PC muscle, you should be able to stop and start the flow of urine mid-stream. If this is difficult, your PC muscle is weak. It may sting a little at first when you stop the flow of urine. This is completely normal and should stop within a few weeks. If it continues you may have an infection, in which case you should see a doctor and clear up the infection before continuing with this and other practices in the book. As with any other muscle that you begin to strengthen, the PC muscle may be a little sore at first. As with all exercises, begin gradually.

The most important part of the practice is simply to start and stop urinating as many times as possible.

Exercise 1

STOPPING THE STREAM

1. INHALE: As you get ready to urinate, inhale deeply.

2. EXHALE AND PUSH OUT: Exhale slowly and forcefully push out the urine. (Clenching your teeth will intensify the practice.)

3. INHALE AND CONTRACT YOUR PC: Inhale and contract your PC muscle to stop the flow of urine midstream.

4. EXHALE AND PUSH OUT AGAIN: Exhale and start urinating again.

5. REPEAT UNTIL FINISHED: Repeat steps 3 and 4 (urinating as you exhale and stopping the stream as you inhale) three to six times or until you have finished going to the bathroom.

To begin, push out your urine as if you are in a hurry and trying to finish as quickly as you can. Standing on your toes and clenching your teeth will also intensify your practice, but the most important part of the practice is simply to start and stop urinating as many times as possible.

In *The Multi-Orgasmic Man*, we teach men other exercises for strengthening their PC muscle, which may be helpful. All PC exercises, however, are based on the simple practice of contracting and releasing your PC muscle. Unlike other kinds of weight lifting, these exercises can be done while you are driving, watching television, and even attending business meetings.

Emptying Your Bladder

You should always urinate before self-pleasuring or lovemaking whenever your bladder is full. A full bladder will make you feel like you need to ejaculate and can actually make it more difficult to keep from ejaculating.

DEVELOPING YOUR SEXUAL SENSITIVITY

Sexual strength is only half of the practice. Sexual sensitivity is equally if not more important. By sensitivity, we mean sensitivity not to your partner's sexual arousal, which we will discuss in a later chapter, but to your own. Becoming multi-orgasmic, like becoming a skillful lover, requires that you discover and learn to master your own arousal.

Unlike the old clichéd techniques of trying to delay ejaculation by desensitizing yourself or distracting yourself with baseball trivia, becoming multi-orgasmic actually requires that you increase your sexual sensitivity and focus more directly on your sexual arousal.

> Becoming multi-orgasmic, like becoming a skillful lover, requires that you discover and learn to master your own arousal.

SEXUAL AROUSAL AND SEXUAL ENERGY

Although sexual arousal is a frequent and significant part of our lives, most of us have little understanding of this process. We call this arousal "getting horny" and snicker as if it were some illicit or juvenile experience. In fact, this arousal is the expansion of our sexual energy, and it is essential to our life and health. According to the Tao, each of us needs to feel aroused—to feel our life-giving sexual energy—every day because when we become aroused, our body produces more sexual hormones.

For Taoism and recently for endocrinology, a branch of Western medicine, sexual hormones are important for our overall health; indeed, some might call them the very fountain of youth. (We discuss this in greater depth in chapter 5, "Sexual Healing.") The reason sex sells is that we are drawn to images that stimulate our sexual energy and sexual hormones. It is extremely liberating for multi-orgasmic men to realize that they have access to this rejuvenating sexual energy all day every day.

Once we learn to circulate our sexual energy, as we explain in chapter 3, we no longer have to wait for sexual encounters to have access to it. In addition, we will discover that we can have far greater control over our arousal

> According to the Tao, each of us needs to feel aroused—to feel our life-giving sexual energy—every day because when we become aroused, our bodies produce more sexual hormones.

and sexual energy. From adolescence or even earlier, most men feel that their sexual desire and arousal are beyond their control and that they are often led around by their penis. Once men learn to become multi-orgasmic and to circulate their sexual energy, they are able to cultivate and transform this sexual energy, giving them a whole new sense of freedom to feel sexual energy only when and where they want.

In chapter 3, you will learn how to circulate this sexual energy throughout your body. But first, you need to learn how to become aware of the subtleties of your expanding sexual energy (that is, your arousal rate) and how to control it. When you are able to control your arousal rate, you will easily be able to have multiple orgasms without cresting over into ejaculation. In the previous section, you learned how to apply the brakes using your PC muscle. Now you need to learn how to gauge the speed of your engine so you know when to put on the brakes.

Men discover a whole new sense of freedom to feel sexual energy only when and where they want.

THE STAGES OF AROUSAL

Most men assume that they are either aroused or not aroused. Either they have an erection or they don't, but in fact there are several different stages of arousal and erection that are important to know. Just as you would want to know the gears of your car, it will help you to know the "gears" of your arousal. Your breathing and heart rate are important signs of your arousal— both will speed up as you get aroused—but the most obvious sign of your arousal is the sexual gauge between your legs: your erection.

The Taoists identified four different stages of erection, which they called the four *attainments*:

1. Lengthening
2. Swelling
3. Hardening
4. Heat

In the first stage, the penis starts to elongate, but it has not begun to rise. In the second stage, it starts to widen and rise, but it is not yet hard. (At this stage, it is really not hard enough to enter your partner unless you use the Soft Entry technique we discuss in chapter 8.) In the third stage, the penis becomes erect and hard, but it is not yet hot. In the fourth and final stage, the penis is stiff and hot. It is at this stage that the testicles draw close to the body and prepare to ejaculate. Relaxing your breathing and drawing your sexual energy up and away from your penis (see chapter 3) will help you to remain in the third stage and the beginning fourth stage without crossing the ejaculatory edge at the end of the fourth stage.

CONTROLLING YOUR AROUSAL RATE

The first step in controlling your arousal rate and learning to become multi-orgasmic is learning to control your breathing. Breathing is the basis for all martial arts and meditative practices, and Sexual Kung Fu is no exception. Your breathing is directly connected to your heart rate. If you are breathing quickly, as after exercising or when hyperventilating, your heart rate increases. When you breathe slowly and deeply, your heart rate decreases. As we discussed above, increased heart rate is one part of orgasm, and breathing quickly signals its approach. By learning to slow down and deepen your breathing, you will learn to control your arousal rate and to revel in orgasms without rushing over into ejaculation.

By learning to slow down and deepen your breathing, you will learn to control your arousal rate and to revel in orgasms without rushing over into ejaculation.

DEEP BREATHING

Deep breathing, or "belly" breathing, is essential to our overall health as well as to our sexual control. Breathing is how our body takes in life-giving oxygen and expels carbon dioxide, the body's waste. Because of stress, however, most of us breathe shallowly, inhaling very little oxygen and exhaling very little carbon dioxide. Deep breathing, or belly breathing, is how you breathed when you were young, before stress started to cut your breath short. The Taoists knew that if one wants to stay young, one must imitate children, and breathing is no exception. In the following exercise you will learn to breathe deeply once again, but this time the benefit will be not only better health but also greater pleasure.

When you are close to ejaculating, the ability to breathe deeply and to slow down your heart rate will be essential. Even once you have learned to be multi-orgasmic, don't forget to still breathe deeply. Deep breathing will help you to circulate your sexual energy throughout your body, which will expand your orgasms and reduce any pressure that you experience when you delay or avoid ejaculating.

Finding the Way

Inhale Through Your Nose

When practicing any of the exercises in this book, always inhale through your nose, which filters and warms the air. When you inhale through your mouth, you breathe unfiltered, unwarmed air, which is harder for your body to assimilate.

Exercise 2

BELLY BREATHING FOR MEN

1. SIT: Sit in a comfortable position and relax your shoulders.

2. HANDS ON ABDOMEN: Place your hands on your abdomen just below your belly button.

3. INHALE DEEPLY: Breathe deeply through your nose so that your belly pushes out (as if you have eaten a big meal).

4. EXHALE FULLY: Keeping your chest relaxed, exhale with some force so that your belly goes back in toward your spine. You should feel your penis and testicles pull up slightly.

5. CONTINUE BELLY BREATHING: Inhale and exhale nine, eighteen, or thirty-six times.

Exercises 1 and 2 are simple but essential. While you may want to read on and try the additional exercises, the more you practice these two exercises, the easier the more advanced multi-orgasmic exercises will be.

Learning to Control Ejaculation

It is possible to learn to be multi-orgasmic during lovemaking with a partner, but it is much easier to develop this new skill by yourself. Like all skills, becoming multi-orgasmic takes practice to perfect, and it will be much easier to focus on your rising arousal if you are not worrying about your partner's arousal as well. In addition, it is much easier to develop your PC muscle and to stop in time if you do not also have to worry about interrupting your partner's climax. Eventually, as you learn to become multi-orgasmic, you will simply need to stop momentarily, breathe deeply, and contract your PC muscles to stop yourself from ejaculating. While this is a book written for couples, it will help you both if you put in some solo time.

SOLO SEX AND SOLO CULTIVATION

Studies show that almost all men masturbate—even older and married men. In addition, almost all men feel some guilt about masturbating. If you don't think you have any guilt feelings about masturbating, ask yourself if you would be willing to call out to your partner who had just come home, "Honey, I'm in the bathroom (or bedroom) masturbating. I'll be right out." Most of us would have no problem informing our partner that we were "in the bathroom," the assumption being that we were relieving our bladder or our bowels, but God forbid we should be relieving an equally basic bodily urge.

The shame about masturbation is widespread, especially in Western society, and masturbation has even been called self-abuse. This attitude is so prevalent, in fact, that a U.S. Surgeon General was asked to resign because she said that masturbation "is part of human sexuality."

The Taoists had no guilt about masturbation. As we have mentioned, for Taoists sex is about medicine and health, not morality. In fact, the Taoists called masturbation *solo cultivation* or *genital exercise* and considered it an important part of learning to control ejaculation and to circulate life-giving sexual energy.

Masturbation, or solo cultivation, can be a satisfying complement to partnered sex and, if you learn to have orgasms without ejaculating, an energizing one as well. As we will discuss in the final chapter, it can also help if your partner is not in the mood or is less often in the mood than you are.

We have two important suggestions regarding learning to self-cultivate:

1. *Make love to yourself.* As we will explain in chapter 6, sexual energy just expands whatever emotions you are feeling. If you are feeling love when you arouse yourself, your expanding sexual energy will increase your love. If you are feeling anger or loneliness when you arouse yourself, your expanding sexual energy will also increase your anger or loneliness. So enter into solo cultivation with a feeling of love and joy at the opportunity to bring such life-giving pleasure to yourself, and the sexual energy will expand this love and joy.

In addition, cultivating your sexual energy while you are feeling love and kindness will make it much easier to control your ejaculation. It is much harder to control your ejaculation if you are feeling anger or impatience.

2. *Take your time.* The longer you are able to solo cultivate and prolong ejaculation, the faster you will be able to learn to become multi-orgasmic.

The Taoists called masturbation *solo cultivation* or *genital exercise* and considered it an important part of learning to control ejaculation and to circulate life-giving sexual energy.

Hartman and Fithian, the pioneering sex researchers who have tested numerous multi-orgasmic men, concluded that if a man can learn to masturbate for fifteen or twenty minutes, he can make love for as long as he wants with his partner. Learning to be patient with yourself will allow you to have patience when you are with your partner.

Once you learn to separate orgasm from ejaculation in this chapter and to circulate sexual energy through your body in chapter 3, you will be able to experience waves of orgasmic pleasure and to circulate that energy through your body. As one multi-orgasmic man described it: "It's something between masturbation and meditation."

Keep in mind that the length of time you solo cultivate should depend on your mood and the moment. As with all lovemaking, there is no right quantity. Everything is about quality. (For additional suggestions and techniques on the Tao of masturbation, please refer to *The Multi-Orgasmic Man*, pp. 41–48.)

Solo cultivation is something between masturbation and meditation.

COOLING DOWN

Now that you have learned to control your PC muscle and your breathing, you have learned the two essential steps for becoming multi-orgasmic. Still, there are other techniques that will help to cool you down when you feel as if you might boil over.

Stop before the point of no return. It is of course better to stop too soon than too late, but most men when they start will need to stop ten to twenty seconds before the point of no return.

Press your penis or your perineum. Pressing the tip or base of your penis with your thumb and fingers (see illustration on p. 17) can decrease your urge to ejaculate. This helps to focus your attention, which can help to concentrate the expanding energy. This is obviously awkward during lovemaking. A more convenient technique during lovemaking is reaching behind you and pressing on your perineum. This will help to focus your attention and interrupt the ejaculatory reflex. Pressing anywhere on the perineum lightly can help, but pressing the famous Million Dollar Point is most effective. This spot is so called because it cost a million dollars (or at the time a million gold pieces) to have a Taoist master show you where it is. The Million Dollar Point is just in front of the anus but before the root of the penis, which extends behind the testicles (see p. 9).

Breathe. When you approach the point of no return, you will need to breathe in deeply, as you have practiced in Exercise 2. Obviously, when you are close to ejaculating, you will breathe in much more quickly. Holding your breath for several seconds until the urge to ejaculate subsides will also

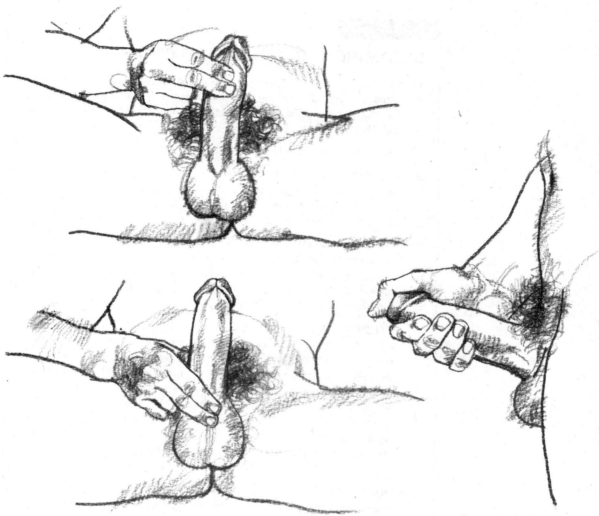

Pressing the head or base of the penis with thumb and fingers can decrease a man's urge to ejaculate.

help immensely. This deep breath helps to contain the expanding sexual energy. Alternatively, quick, shallow breaths can help to disperse the sexual energy. See which works best for you.

Contract your PC *muscle.* Once again, your PC muscle surrounds your prostate, through which your semen must pass during the expulsion phase of orgasm. When you squeeze your prostate during contractile-phase orgasm (when it is contracting involuntarily), you can stop yourself from cresting over from contraction (orgasm) to expulsion (ejaculation).

BECOMING A MULTI-ORGASMIC MAN

1. LUBRICATE: Start by lubricating your penis. (Lubrication, as you may already know, will increase your sensations and make it possible to solo cultivate longer. Oil is generally better than lotion, which dries up more quickly.)

2. SELF-PLEASURE: Self-pleasure however you like.

3. PAY ATTENTION TO YOUR AROUSAL: Pay close attention to your arousal rate. Once again, try to notice your increasing levels of arousal: notice the tingling at the root of your penis, notice the stages of erection, notice your breathing change and your heart rate increase.

4. BREATHE AND CONTRACT YOUR PC MUSCLE: As you feel yourself getting close to the point of no return, stop, breathe deeply, and lightly contract your PC muscle around your prostate. You can press on your penis or perineum, but your breath and your PC muscle are the most important, as is stopping in time.

5. FEEL ORGASMIC CONTRACTIONS IN YOUR PELVIS: Continue to pleasure yourself, coming increasingly close to the point of no return. If non-arousal is 0 and ejaculation is 10.0, then orgasm is at 9.8, so go slow. Start and stop, arousing yourself more and more (9.0, 9.1, and so on), and let yourself fall back into a contractile-phase orgasm without falling forward into an ejaculation. Notice the involuntary contraction of your prostate (and anus) that occurs during contractile-phase orgasm. Remember that these prostate orgasms may feel like mini-orgasms at first. Eventually they will be indistinguishable from ejaculatory orgasms, but you need to walk before you can run.

6. ENJOY: After you have peaked several times without ejaculating, stop. You will feel peaceful and/or energized afterward. You may even notice the sexual energy starting to rise in your body as tingling or prickling in your torso or head. This is completely natural and the beginning of transforming your genital orgasms into whole-body orgasms.

It may take you a few times before you can feel the contractile-phase orgasms without cresting over into ejaculation, but don't worry; with a little practice and a little patience you will soon be having multiple orgasms that are as intense and as pleasurable as any ejaculatory orgasm.

Pelvic Pressure

Pressure in your pelvic area is a natural result of the increased blood flow and sexual energy in your genital area. If the pressure feels uncomfortable, you can simply ejaculate, or you can breathe deeply (as described in Exercise 2) as well as massaging your perineum and testicles gently. This will help your body to assimilate this powerful and healing energy. In chapter 3, you will learn to circulate this energy out of your genitals and to the rest of your body.

Your Prostate

When a man gets aroused, the prostate naturally enlarges slightly. By contracting your PC muscle around your prostate during and after self-pleasuring or lovemaking you will not only help control ejaculation, you will also help reduce any pressure on your prostate.

These PC contractions will also guide the energy out of your pelvis and up your body (see chapter 3). This will further reduce the pressure on the prostate gland and testicles. You can also massage the perineum, testicles, and tailbone to help relieve pressure and disperse the built-up sexual energy.

If you feel a burning sensation when you urinate or prolonged pelvic pain, you may have a urinary tract infection. You should see a physician and clear this up before trying or continuing with the practice. While trying to get rid of the infection, you will need to ejaculate more regularly.

WHEN TO STOP

Most men stop masturbating or having sex when they ejaculate. Once you become multi-orgasmic, this obvious end point will no longer exist. You will therefore need to decide when you and your partner are satisfied. On some days you will want a quick sexual experience, and on others you will want leisurely lovemaking. Your needs will change based on your mood and the moment.

When you begin to be multi-orgasmic during lovemaking, it is important that you give yourself and your partner time to adjust. You do not want to turn sex into a chore or an endurance test for you or her. So talk to your partner, and let both of your desire determine the duration of your lovemaking. The more she cultivates her own PC muscle and sexual desire, the better matched the two of you will be.

Your PC muscle is like any other muscle—it strengthens with use—but as with all exercise, you don't want to push it too far too fast. Also, if you are solo or duo cultivating for more than twenty minutes, which you often may once you are multi-orgasmic, it is important to let your erection decrease somewhat about every twenty minutes to allow the blood to recirculate through your body.

It is important to let your erection decrease somewhat about every twenty minutes to allow the blood to recirculate through your body.

WHEN TO EJACULATE

According to the Taoists, pleasure was not the only reason to become multi-orgasmic. They also believed that multiple orgasms were healthy and healing for the body. The more orgasms a man had without ejaculating, the more sexual energy he could circulate through his body. While orgasms, for the Taoists, are energizing, ejaculations are depleting. While there is nothing wrong with ejaculating from time to time, the Taoists felt that as a man got older ejaculating too often could physically exhaust him. The Taoists linked many erection problems to this physical exhaustion. (If you have difficulty getting or maintaining an erection, you may wish to read "Snake Charming: Overcoming Impotence" in *The Multi-Orgasmic Man.*)

If you are very young, you may not have experienced the depletion that often follows ejaculation, but most men after they ejaculate are tired or want to go to sleep. (We discuss the Taoist and medical views on the topic in detail in chapter 5, "Sexual Healing.")

According to the Taoists, each time you have an orgasm (without ejaculating), you draw more energy into your body. Therefore, if you eventually do ejaculate, you lose less of your energy. This is why ejaculation after multiple orgasms is less draining than the old "wham, bam, thank you, Ma'am" ejaculation. If you have half a dozen orgasms and then ejaculate, you will lose approximately half as much energy.

The Taoists recommended that each man ejaculate according to his own condition depending on his age, his health, and the circumstances of his life. If you are getting sick or working hard, you will want to conserve more energy. During the winter, you, like all of nature, will also want to conserve more energy. However, if you are on vacation, you may want to ejaculate more. Of course, if you are trying to conceive a child, you will need to ejaculate whenever your partner is ovulating. Sun Ssu-miao, one of the leading physicians of ancient China, recommended that, overall, a man can attain good health and longevity by ejaculating twice a month.

Sun Ssu-miao also offered more specific guidelines by which one could decide how often to ejaculate:

A man of *twenty* can ejaculate once every *four* days.
A man of *thirty* can ejaculate once every *eight* days.
A man of *forty* can ejaculate once every *ten* days.
A man of *fifty* can ejaculate once every *twenty* days.
A man of *sixty* should not ejaculate.

Of course, a man of any age can continue to have sex and have multiple non-ejaculatory orgasms. Indeed, the Taoists believed there is no reason that men and women shouldn't have sex until the day they die. While you may worry about the decrease in the number of ejaculations or the prohibition on them after sixty, once you experience multiple non-ejaculatory orgasms, the typical "squirt" orgasm is a pale comparison and hardly missed.

The most important thing, however, is not to give yourself a hard time about ejaculating. When you feel that you are past the point of no return and are going to ejaculate, enjoy it. Many men who want to practice Healing Love start to judge themselves if they have trouble learning to control their ejaculations. Focus on being with your partner and exchanging Healing Love, not on whether you did or did not ejaculate.

Learning to circulate your sexual energy (as you will learn in chapter 3) can happen even if you eventually ejaculate. This will far reduce the feeling of depletion after ejaculation. In addition, after you do ejaculate, you can also contract your PC muscle to tighten your pelvic muscles and reduce the amount of energy that is lost.

In the end, what is most important is that you are making love with yourself and with your partner. Cultivating compassion for yourself and for your partner is much more important than how much energy you conserve.

From Genital Orgasms to Whole-Body Orgasms

The physical techniques described in this chapter, especially breathing and contracting your PC muscle, will allow you to separate orgasm from ejaculation

> A man can attain good health and longevity by ejaculating twice a month.

and become multi-orgasmic. Still, the real secret to long-term ejaculatory control—and multiple orgasms—is learning to circulate your sexual energy out of your genitals and to the rest of your body. As long as sexual energy continues to build up in your genitals, it will eventually cause you to ejaculate unless you stop lovemaking or learn to redirect it out of your genitals. Ejaculation can happen only if there is enough energy and blood in the genitals to trigger ejaculation.

By drawing the energy up and away from your genitals, as we explain in chapter 3, you will be able to control your sexual energy for as long as you want. Conserving and circulating the energy magnifies the intensity of the orgasm and enables the body to retain the energy for longer-lasting pleasure and health.

The combination of a man's using his sexual strength (his PC muscle), his sexual sensitivity (his ability to be aware of his arousal rate), and his ability to circulate sexual energy should help immeasurably in allowing him to become multi-orgasmic.

Women lose far less energy than men when they orgasm (and even when they ejaculate[6]). However, when women have a single strong terminal orgasm, they often experience a loss of energy and a loss of their desire to make love. By drawing their sexual energy up and multiplying their orgasms, they will feel more energized and more aroused. This is particularly important for women who have difficulty feeling desire

Both you and your partner will be able to expand your genital orgasms into whole-body orgasms as you learn to circulate the energy and pleasure to the rest of your body. This is also the basis for transforming that wonderful orgasmic twitch into an experience that is ecstatic, healing, intimate, and for some even spiritual. The rest of the Arts of the Bedchamber await you.

Conserving and circulating the energy magnifies the intensity of the orgasm and enables the body to retain the energy for longer-lasting pleasure and health.

CHAPTER 2

The Pool of Desire: Multiple Orgasms for Women

In this chapter, you will discover:

- The Power of Your Desire and How to Exercise Your Passion

- Your Erotic Fingerprint

- How to Strengthen Your PC Muscle for Stronger Orgasms

- The Nine Steps to Multiple Orgasms for Any Woman

- How to Overcome Difficulties Having Orgasms

Every woman can have a passionate and deeply satisfying sex life. Many women, however, still have difficulty experiencing their full desire and being regularly orgasmic. According to one recent study that we discuss below, one-third of women experience orgasm only occasionally and another third do not experience orgasm at all. If you are one of these women, this chapter will help you reach your true orgasmic and multi-orgasmic potential.

If you are a woman who already experiences pleasure and orgasms easily, this chapter and the next will help you to intensify the pleasure and orgasms you already enjoy. Even if you are already multi-orgasmic, we strongly encourage you to take the time to read and do the exercises in this chapter. The messages we receive as women about our bodies, our desire, and our pleasure are so pervasive it is difficult to embrace our sexual selves fully. This chapter will help you cultivate your potential for even more profound pleasure and intimacy.

Desire Is the Energy of Life

Desire is not just the impulse that leads us to the bedroom; it is the pulse that keeps us alive.

Desire is not just the impulse that leads us to the bedroom; it is the pulse that keeps us alive. Sexual desire is related to the desire that motivates us in all other aspects of our life. For Taoists, sexual energy, or *ching*, is an essential part of our total physical energy, called *chi*. People who are in touch with their sexual energy will have more energy to pursue their goals and dreams in the rest of their lives. In chapter 3 we will discuss in detail how to cultivate your sexual energy and how to transform it to increase your overall energy. But first we begin by focusing on your current level of desire and pleasure so that you can learn to enhance them both.

PRIORITIZING PLEASURE

While we all have the potential for enormous desire and great passion, we face obstacles that make it difficult to experience them. The demands of work, friends, and family keep most of us busier than we'd like to be. Lovemaking often gets put off until bedtime, when we must choose between intimacy or much-needed sleep. In a recent in-depth study of more than 12,000 couples, the authors concluded that fatigue was the greatest obstacle to satisfying sex.[1] For our sexual life to flourish, we need to make our pleasure a priority.

For our sexual life to flourish, we need to make our pleasure a priority.

There is a widely held assumption among women that our sexuality and desire are not nearly as important as the other priorities in our life: our partner, our children, our work, our home. It is difficult for us to make our personal well-being a priority in any sphere of our life and particularly when it is something as self-focused as our own pleasure. But just as the other spheres of our life affect our sexuality, our sexuality can positively affect every other aspect of our life. A sexually satisfied woman is much happier and more optimistic, not to mention a better partner, mother, or worker.

Like anything truly worthwhile, sexuality requires that we prioritize it and make time for it. Just as we need to dedicate time for our family and our job, we need to dedicate time each week away from phones, children, or other demands in order to nurture our sexual self. We would never expect our body to be in shape without exercising regularly. The same is true with our sexuality. To have a healthy sex life, we need to exercise our passion regularly.

THE BEAUTY IDEAL

Another common obstacle to desire for many women is the feeling that we are not attractive enough to be desirable or even to experience our own desire. Our society often conveys that there is only one kind of beautiful female body: an unrealistically thin one with large breasts. How unfortunate that the barrage of media images of airbrushed women's bodies has made us lose sight of the fact that every body is unique and beautiful. And even more to the point, every body, no matter what size and shape, is capable of giving and receiving pleasure.

We are enormously influenced by the body images we see on TV shows and posters and in magazines and cosmetics advertisements. Medically speaking, most models are far below their optimum body weight. It is also important to remember that these "ideal" images are relative within time and culture. Female movie stars and models fifty years ago in the United States weighed on average 20 percent more than they do now and were much closer to their optimum body weight.

Within other cultures many different body types (large breasts or small breasts, large lips or small lips, large hips or small hips) are revered. It is our curves that make us womanly, and most men (and women) prefer a lot more flesh on their partners than the media portray. Later in this chapter, we will get to know and love our body as an integral part of increasing our desire and our pleasure.

> Just as the other spheres of our life affect our sexuality, our sexuality can positively affect every other aspect of our life. A sexually satisfied woman is much happier and more optimistic, not to mention a better partner, mother, or worker.

> Every body, no matter what size and shape, is capable of giving and receiving pleasure.

Building Desire: Exploring Your Erotic Potential

The first step toward multiple orgasms and a more satisfying sexual life lies in increasing our powers of desire. In the following exercises, you will explore your erotic potential. This exercise is useful no matter how much desire you currently experience.

For those of you who worry that you have "too much" desire, you should know that the Taoists considered having strong desire to be a great blessing and a wellspring of energy for cultivating our physical, emotional, and spiritual life. While sexual desire can be distracting (and even annoying) when it is unsatisfied or unable to be expressed, learning to mobilize this energy for your benefit will transform your life. Increased sexual energy, or *ching*, can be transformed into physical energy, or *chi*, for improving our body's health and well-being. The more desire and energy we have, the more vitality we can experience. The Healing Love practice will give you access to your sexual energy when and where you want and will allow you to channel any remaining sexual energy into your creative, emotional, and spiritual life. We will demonstrate how to transform our sexual energy in chapter 3.

If you find that you consistently have more desire than your partner, you will want to encourage him to read this book and *The Multi-Orgasmic Man*. When men learn to become multi-orgasmic (without ejaculating), they find that they have a great deal more sexual desire and are much more able to satisfy their partners. Men are also often distracted by work and other pressures, so it is important for both of you to take time to focus on your sexual life away from these other demands.

Most of us are strongly influenced by the attitudes about sexuality we encountered as children. The comfort or discomfort with bodily pleasure of the adults around us sent strong messages about the value of desire and sexuality. What kind of model did your parents or other adults in your life provide of a committed, sexual relationship?

In addition to providing models of a sexual relationship, parents have varying attitudes toward the sensual and sexual potential of their growing children. Consider the role of touch in your family. Was there lots of jovial hugging or very little physical contact? Did you experience touch as welcome affection or was it sometimes uncomfortable?

In addition to our family, the wider cultural attitudes regarding sexuality also have a lasting influence on our sexuality. Whether we accept these attitudes or rebel against them, they still shape our sexual selves.

Our sexuality grows out of our unique sexual history, the situations and

YOUR EROTIC FINGERPRINT

Answer each of these questions for yourself as a means to understanding your unique sexuality. You may wish to write down the answers to these questions, or you may wish to simply answer them in your head. It might be helpful to start a journal to explore your sexual self through the exercises presented in this book. This journal need not be shared with anyone, not even your partner, unless you wish to do so.

As a child:

1. What were the attitudes about sexuality and about bodies in your family as you were growing up?

2. What was your first sexual experience like? Was it alone or with another person?

3. How have these experiences influenced your current views of your body and your sexual life?

As an adult:

1. At what moments in your life do you recall feeling the most desire or pleasure?

2. What places, times of day, or partners have aroused you the most?

3. In what specific ways were these moments different from and similar to those in your life now?

And now:

1. In your current life, what things increase or decrease your desire?

2. If you could create the perfect erotic situation for yourself, what would it look like? (Do not limit your imagination here. Your fantasy life does not need to have any relationship to your present life. There is no greater generator of desire than an active imagination.)

Exploring your sexual history will help you discover your individual erotic fingerprint.

experiences that we found sexy as we were growing up. Exploring your sexual history will help you discover your individual erotic fingerprint.

What have you rediscovered about yourself? Can you harness the desires of your past to fuel your present life and relationships? Once you have "found" your desire, whether you felt it in the past or in a real or imagined present, the desire is yours. You can bring that desire into your current life through the power of your imagination. While doing the exercises in this chapter, recreate for yourself those specific situations (whether historical fact or future fantasy) that get you hot. You may actually be able to do this in the privacy of your home, but more likely you will need to use your memory and imagination.

By exploring your erotic fingerprint you're opening up your intimate past. Our sexual history can be a great erotic resource, but most of us have difficult and even painful memories of our sexual past that can interfere with our satisfaction in the present. Exploring and understanding our past takes the power from these negative memories and reclaims it for our present. We strongly encourage you to explore and share these experiences with a trusted partner, friend, or therapist. If this does not seem possible, try drawing, painting, or writing about these experiences. The more you are able to shed the light of your current mature understanding on the shadows of the past, the less hold these experiences will have on you and the more you can revel in the sexuality of the present.

EVERYDAY EROS

One of the secrets of desire is that it starts long before we reach the bedroom. Poets the world over have known that the path to lovemaking is as important as the destination. While each woman has her own erotic fingerprint, many of us share certain images and situations that increase our desire. Many women find that increasing the sensual nature of their everyday life helps keep their body alive to their sensual and sexual potential.

It is important to nurture this aspect of yourself in whatever way you find helpful: wearing clothes that caress your body, smelling candles, flowers, and other scents in the house, listening to sensual music, taking hot baths by candlelight, or eating foods that you find tantalizing. According to the Tao, women are energized by beauty. By bringing beauty and sensuality into your everyday life, you expand your desire and your overall sense of joy.

Be alive to the erotic possibility of the world around you. Notice the beautiful diversity of bodies all around you. If you are able to look at and appreciate other women's bodies without judging them, you will be able to accept your own body for its own unique and beautiful form.

Open yourself to the erotic possibilities of art and nature. Let yourself dance to beautiful music, or feel the wind on your body and let it stir you. Be open to the world around you, not to appeal to someone else but to pleasure yourself. Discovering the erotic possibilities of our life gives us incredible power. For the Tao, our sexual energy is the very foundation of our being and is essential for being fully alive.

This exploration of your desire is a process that can be life transforming. It is a great new adventure that you are embarking on. As with any other knowledge

According to the Tao, women are energized by beauty. By bringing beauty and sensuality into your everyday life, you expand your desire and your overall sense of joy.

or skill that you acquire, the more time that you spend, the more you will get out of it. The small amounts of time you invest in your sexual potential will result in tremendous rewards—in the pleasure you receive, in the deeper relationship you have with your partner, in the increased joy in your life, and in your greater overall vitality.

Knowing Your Body

Now that we have begun kindling our desire, it is time to embrace and explore our bodies. Unfortunately, for many women, looking at our naked body is filled with anxiety. Women have been learning for years to evaluate their body in comparison to impossible bodily ideals. The Tao recognized that when we celebrate ideal images, we make all others feel inadequate.

While you are engaged in pursuing your orgasmic potential, try to take a holiday from body criticism. Do your best not to engage in complaints or worries about your body alone or with others. It is amazing how difficult this can be! Try to remember that a judged and criticized body does not yield pleasure nearly as easily as a body that is loved and appreciated. As we look at ourselves and touch ourselves, we start the process of loving ourselves.

Find a mirror that is as near to full length as possible. Again, you will need freedom from interruption and soft lighting.

> The small amounts of time you invest in your sexual potential will result in tremendous rewards—in the pleasure you receive, in the deeper relationship you have with your partner, in the increased joy in your life, and in your greater overall vitality.

> A judged and criticized body does not yield pleasure nearly as easily as a body that is loved and appreciated.

Exercise 5

LOVING YOUR BODY

1. TAKE IT FROM THE TOP: Start at the top of your head and move downward, noticing the particular artistry of your body. Notice the color, shape, and texture of your hair, the color of your eyes, and the shape of your face. Note how soft your lips are compared with your cheeks. Notice your ears and your neck, the length of your arms.

2. NO BODY CRITICS: Whenever negative thoughts occur to you, such as, "The backs of my arms are flabby," take a moment to verbally appreciate that part of your body for what it does. For example, thank your arms for the great job they do at lifting, writing, and hugging.

3. APPRECIATE EACH PART: Find something kind to say about each part of your body. As you move down your body, appreciate the particular shape of your breasts, the color of your nipples, the soft curves of your belly and hips, your buttocks, the roundness of your thighs, the length of your legs, the stability of your feet. Every woman's body is uniquely beautiful. You can feel desire and be desired exactly as you are.

Most of us are familiar with the shape and size of our hands since we see them every day, but very few of us are as familiar with the size and shape of our sexual anatomy. In order to pleasure yourself or to show your partner how to pleasure you, it will help if you are familiar with your body's erogenous zones. If you have never seen what your genitals look like, we strongly encourage you to take a few minutes to look at them.

Find some private time when you will not be interrupted. Lie back, preferably on a bed or a couch, prop yourself up with pillows, and use a hand mirror in front of your genitals until you can easily see them. If you lean the mirror against a pillow, you may be able to use a flashlight or other direct lighting to see better.

Getting Up Close and Personal—a mirror can help a woman become familiar with her own sexual anatomy.

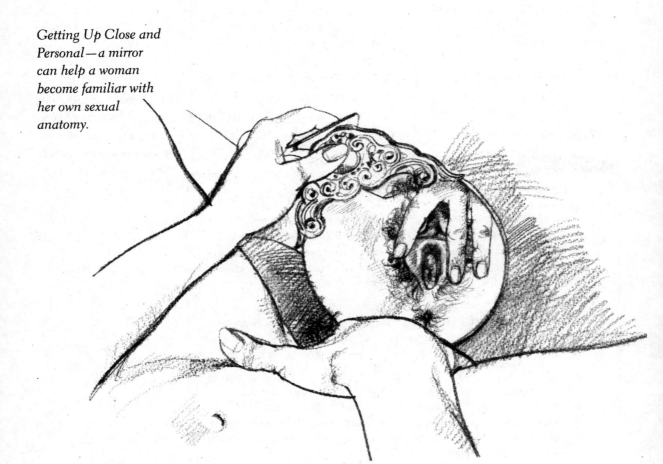

GETTING UP CLOSE AND PERSONAL

1. YOUR OUTER LIPS: Place the mirror between your legs so that you can see your genitals. You'll notice that the thicker, outer, lips (or labia majora) are covered with hair on the outside. If you part these, you will see the smaller lips of the vagina (or labia minora), which have no hair.

2. YOUR CLITORIS: Part the inner lips and look at the top, where the lips meet (or at twelve o'clock on a clock face, if you are looking in your mirror). There you will see your clitoris, a half-centimeter bump. You will notice (and you will need good lighting for this) that there is some tissue, often called the hood, surrounding the clitoris that can be withdrawn in order to see the clitoris itself.

3. YOUR VAGINA: If you move directly downward (that is, toward your anus) you will find your urethra, a sometimes-difficult-to-spot small opening below the clitoris. This is where your urine comes out when you pee. Another centimeter or two down is the vagina. Often the opening of the vagina is covered with folds of tissue. If you bear down as if you are going to have a bowel movement, you will notice that the tissue opens up, usually showing you the entrance to the vagina, which extends into your body like a canal.

4. YOUR CERVIX: The only accessible part of your sexual anatomy you won't be able to see during this bodily exploration is your cervix. Though you can't see your cervix without the help of a speculum (a device that props open the vagina), you can certainly feel your cervix. If you place one or two fingers within your vagina all the way to the back and bear down as if you're having a bowel movement, you will touch something that feels like the end of your nose. This is your cervix.

5. YOUR PERINEUM: Below the vagina you will notice that the inner lips join together in a very muscular area that is covered with normal skin and sometimes hair, called the perineum.

6. YOUR ANUS: At the bottom of the perineum you can see your anus, which is a puckered circular area of skin with a strong muscle inside.

Now that you have seen your own genitals, it might be helpful to know some general facts about this most personal and often mysterious part of our body.

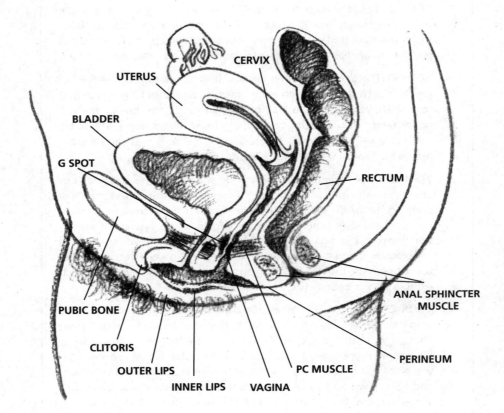

Woman's sexual anatomy

Outer Lips: While all women have pubic hair, the color, texture, and amount are different. In general vaginal lips are pale pink, red, dark tan, or brown, depending on your skin color. In most women, they can be quite irregular in shape, and all shapes and sizes are completely normal. During increased arousal, both the outer and inner lips become swollen with blood, much as a man's penis becomes engorged during sexual arousal. In fact, the female outer lips and the male shaft of the penis start out as the same tissue in the early development of the fetus. These tissues can be very sensitive if gently stroked during sexual play.

Clitoris: The clitoris is the anatomical equivalent of the head of the penis in a man and has just as many nerve endings as the head of the penis, only concentrated into a much smaller space. This makes it the most sensitive sexual organ in either sex. It is also the only organ in either sex exclusively dedicated to sexual pleasure. The naked clitoris is exquisitely tender, and most women prefer more indirect stimulation, either through the surrounding skin, from the side, or through the hood. The clitoris swells during sexual arousal and becomes much more prominent.

Vagina: The vagina is normally well lubricated from the glands that exist at its entrance. Almost all women have some normal clear, whitish, or yellowish discharge from the vagina at all times. This is normal and is the vagina's way of cleaning itself.

Cervix: The cervix is the lower tip of your uterus, which resides at the very back of your vagina. When you menstruate, blood flows through the cervix, and when you give birth, the cervix dilates in order to let the baby out. Some women report that the cervix can be stimulated during sexual intercourse, while others find any pressing against the cervix painful. If you find it painful when your partner's penis hits your cervix, you can simply adjust the angle of penetration.

Perineum: The perineum stretches the centimeter or two between the vagina and the anus and is a collection of muscles forming the floor of the pelvis and supporting all the sexual and pelvic organs. This collection of muscles is called the pubococcygeus (or PC) muscle. Later in the chapter we will talk in more detail about the PC muscle, which is essential for becoming orgasmic and multi-orgasmic. The perineum is sometimes very sensitive to touch and can be sexually arousing.

Anus: The anus, which has many nerve endings, can be extremely sexually arousing for some people. Many of the same nerves that innervate the vagina innervate the rectum as well. Most women prefer to be significantly aroused before touching this area, although some women experience great sensitivity in this area at all times.

You may be concerned about cleanliness and touching this area. Washing the anus with soap and water before self-pleasuring or lovemaking may be a good idea if you plan to touch there. We would recommend not using any soap on the vaginal area, however, because it can be irritating.

Also remember that you never want to touch the anal area and then directly touch the vaginal area without washing hands or other sexual objects first. It is important not to let bacteria from the anus enter or come near the vagina, which has its own natural bacteria. Using latex gloves, condoms, or dental dams for stimulation solves that problem nicely since one is able to dispose of them after anal stimulation. (In short, anything that goes in the anus needs to be washed before it goes in the vagina.)

Pleasuring Yourself

There are many taboos in our society against a woman stimulating herself sexually, although these have lessened somewhat over the past twenty years. Fifty years ago, about a third of women had masturbated by age twenty. Now the number is closer to half.

Still, many women feel apprehensive or guilty about touching themselves or masturbating. Other women can't live without it! Whatever your own feelings, you should be aware that every leading sex expert believes that masturbation is absolutely vital to increasing sexual pleasure alone *and* with a partner. There is no better way to find out where and how you like to be touched or pleasured. There is in fact no better way to improve your lovemaking and to help your partner satisfy you than to know intimately your own sexual landscape.

Some women fear that masturbation will decrease their desire to make love with their partner. In fact, the reverse is true. In general the more sexually active and aware of your body you are, the more you will want to be sexual with a loving partner.

Masturbation does not take the place of partnered lovemaking but offers a creative and wonderful alternative to partnered lovemaking. This means that neither partner is completely dependent on the other for satisfying sexual needs. This gives both partners the freedom to say yes and to say no to lovemaking, without leaving their partner high and dry sexually.

In Healing Love and in the meditative practices of Taoist sexuality, masturbation is referred to as self-cultivation. In these practices you awaken your sexual energy and then are able to transform and store it in your body for greater vitality and longevity. We'll explore this in great detail in chapter 3. You first need to discover the paths to self-pleasure before you can learn to solo cultivate.

For the Body Exploration exercise you will need at least thirty minutes when you will not be interrupted. The room should be comfortable and feel intimate and private. You may want to adjust lighting, music, and bedding to get the feel you like. If you desire lubrication, you can use a natural oil (almond or olive) or a water-soluble lubricant. Newer, thinner lubricants, such as Bodywise Liquid Silk, are easiest to handle and most like your natural secretions.

There is in fact no better way to improve your lovemaking and to help your partner to satisfy you than to know intimately your own sexual landscape.

In Healing Love and in the meditative practices of Taoist sexuality, masturbation is referred to as self-cultivation.

You should feel no pressure to bring yourself to orgasm during this exploration. The point is to become familiar with what your body likes. If you find yourself moving toward orgasm, of course that is fine. What follows is a detailed map by which to explore your body and find your pleasure spots. You may want to read through it once before beginning the exercise. Feel free to follow the lead of your own pleasure.

For some of us, touching ourselves can induce feelings of anxiety. This is understandable given the negative attitudes about self-touch in our society. However, nothing can cool the warmth of pleasure faster than the chill of fear.

At the beginning of each exercise in this chapter and at any time that you feel anxious, we suggest that you practice belly breathing. The Taoists have used this deep breathing practice for millennia to calm the mind and spread healing energy throughout the body. It is also similar to deep breathing exercises recommended clinically by many health practitioners for stress relief and relaxation.

Exercise 7

BELLY BREATHING FOR WOMEN

1. SIT: Sit in a comfortable position and relax your shoulders.

2. HANDS ON ABDOMEN: Place your hands on your abdomen just below your belly button.

3. INHALE DEEPLY: Breathe deeply through your nose so that your belly pushes out (as if you have eaten a big meal).

4. EXHALE FULLY: Keeping your chest relaxed, exhale with some force so that your belly goes back in toward your spine.

5. CONTINUE BELLY BREATHING: Inhale and exhale nine times, feeling your body relax. Acknowledge the thoughts that pass through your mind and then let them go. Do not dwell upon any particular thought, but only observe it and let it pass. Practice this until you are able to observe your thoughts without having any emotional reaction to them.

BODY EXPLORATION

1. RELAX: Sit or lie in a comfortable position.

2. BREATHE: Take nine deep breaths to relax your mind and body.

3. YOUR HEAD: Start by running your fingers through your hair, feeling the sensation on your scalp with your soft fingertips or with your nails. Move your fingers over your face, feeling the curves of your cheekbones and your lips. Some women find their ears to be very erotic. Try circling your earlobes, putting fingers inside, pulling on the lobes, or stroking the skin around your ears.

4. YOUR NECK: Move your hands down your neck, noting how it feels to be touched at the nape of your neck in the back, and in the front as your neck joins with your chest. Where are the spots that are particularly sensitive or responsive for you?

5. YOUR ARMS: Move down each of your shoulders and along your arms. You might find that the inside of your arms is very sensitive, as are your armpits. Hands and fingers can also be very sensitive, particularly the skin between your fingers. The body is excited by a variety of sensations. If you wish, you can try licking or sucking parts of your hands, fingers, or arms and then blowing on them. You can also use feathers or soft cloths to draw across your skin for more stimulation.

6. YOUR BREASTS: Hold your breasts in your hands. Circle around the outsides of your breasts, feeling how soft the skin is. Some women like to have their breasts squeezed. Others prefer a very light touch. Move in slowly toward your nipples. For many women the nipples are exquisitely sensitive to stimulation. Experiment with light touch and with harder pressure or squeezing the nipples. In general the more a woman is aroused, the more intense the stimulation of the breast or nipples can be. Most women like to begin with a softer touch. See what feels best to you.

7. YOUR BELLY: Next stroke down your belly and feel where it curves. A soft belly is considered extremely sensual in most parts of the world. This is why belly dancing is so erotic. Touch and explore your navel.

8. YOUR BUTTOCKS: Use your fingernails to stroke down your back and your buttocks. Cup your buttocks in your hands and feel their solid weight.

9. YOUR LEGS: Now move down to your toes. The feet can be very sensitive, particularly along the arch and between the toes. Some lovers enjoy sucking on each other's toes. Using the oil, run your fingers between your toes. Touch the arch of your foot and the back of your heel. Now massage up your calves, feeling the muscles underneath. The backs of the knees are sensitive and sometimes ticklish. Move up along the outside and then the inside of your thighs. As you move up closer to your pubic triangle you'll notice that the skin of the thighs gets more sensitive and softer.

10. YOUR PUBIC TRIANGLE: Run your fingers through your pubic hair. Feel the softness and fullness of your outer vaginal lips. With one hand, open the outer lips and with the other hand explore the inner lips of your vagina. You may find oil or lubricant useful in keeping yourself lubricated and comfortable. Touch the area around your

vagina and your perineum. Where is the skin most sensitive?

11. YOUR CLITORIS: Move your fingers around your clitoris. Many women like somewhat indirect pressure from the side or above their clitoris. Experiment with different strokes, pressure from the sides, circling around the clitoris, gentle pinching, rhythmic pressure versus constant pressure, a light touch versus a firmer touch. Remember that the point is to explore and not necessarily to have an orgasm.

12. YOUR VAGINA: Move your fingers down to your vagina. Using oil or lubricant if needed, place one finger inside your vagina. Notice that it is slightly tighter when you first go in and then opens up somewhat. The tighter area is your PC (pubococcygeus) muscle, which we will discuss below. The vagina is amazingly elastic so that it can fit close around one finger or around four fingers or around a large penis or dildo. Explore the different walls of the vagina and note their different textures and sensations.

13. YOUR G SPOT: Along the front wall of the vagina on the belly side, approximately one-third to two-thirds of a finger length inside, there is an area the size of a dime that can become raised and ridged when you are aroused. This area overlies the famed G spot.[2] Taoists have referred to this spot for thousands of years as the Black Pearl. It is not always easy to find, but most women have better luck when they're aroused and the area is enlarged and more prominent.

Using a hooked finger or dildo, enter the vagina approximately an inch or two and press rhythmically upward toward the belly. The location varies for each woman, so you will need to explore. Stimulation of the G spot often produces a sensation of needing to urinate (because the tissue of the G spot surrounds the urethra). With relaxation and persistence, this urge fades to a pleasurable fullness. Orgasms from this spot feel different from clitoral orgasms, somewhat deeper and more diffuse. With orgasm from G-spot arousal, some women ejaculate through their urethra a clear fluid that is different from urine.[3]

14. YOUR OTHER SPOTS: Some women find they have an X and a Y spot to the left or right of the G spot at the same depth. In addition, some women find that deep in the vagina, either just in front of or just behind the cervix, in the cul-de-sac, a pleasurable sensation is experienced with penetration. Spots such as the G spot or the area just in front of the cervix are more easily stimulated from behind, either with fingers, dildo, or penis. Spots on the back wall of the vagina can be better stimulated from the front, such as in the missionary position. Using your fingers, dildo, or vibrator (or any long smooth object that may be handy!), you can see for yourself where your own pleasurable spots may be.

15. YOUR PERINEUM AND ANUS: Moving downward from the vagina you find the perineum, the muscular bridge between the vagina and the rectum. When aroused, some women find this area stimulating. Even more common is for the anus and the skin around the anus to be sensitive. If you have never touched yourself in this area or been touched pleasurably in this area, start with very light stimulation of the area around the anus. You may want to experiment with penetration (using lots of lubricant) if it is pleasurable for you. Some women do not find this area particularly pleasurable, and you can certainly skip that part of the stimulation if you wish.

If this exercise leaves you titillated and wanting more, forge ahead to the next section, where we explore our orgasmic potential. If you're still feeling shy or uncomfortable, you will want to repeat this exercise a number of times and do belly breathing when necessary. Remember, the more you know about what turns you on, the more pleasure you can experience and ultimately share with your partner. Let this exercise be a catalyst for a lifetime of self-love.

Cultivating Your Orgasmic Potential

One-third of women are not able to have orgasms at all, one-third have orgasms occasionally, and only one-third have orgasms consistently

Now that you have explored your body's sensual terrain, you can learn how to bring yourself to orgasm whenever you want. According to sex researchers Beverly Whipple, William Hartman, and Marilyn Fithian, one-third of women are not able to have orgasms at all, one-third have orgasms occasionally, and only one-third have orgasms consistently.[4] If you are one of the women who orgasms not at all or only occasionally, the exercises in this book will assist you in having as many orgasms as you want, when you want.

THE CLINICAL ORGASM

The experience of orgasm is unique to each person. Particularly for women, the length and intensity of orgasm may vary greatly from person to person. It will also vary from one sexual experience to another and even within the same lovemaking session. With this said, here is the classic description of a single female orgasm, by pioneering sex researchers Masters and Johnson.

Sexual arousal draws blood to the pelvic area, causing swelling of the clitoris and the vaginal lips. With increased stimulation, the woman proceeds through an excitement phase to an orgasm consisting of contractions of the PC muscle, the sling of muscle that surrounds the anus, vagina, and urethra. The contractions are approximately one second each, and the total orgasm lasts from three to twelve seconds.

The woman experiences extreme pleasure and throbbing sensations centered in the pelvic area but radiating outward. During orgasm her rate of breathing, her heart rate, and her muscle tone increase. After the orgasm her arousal declines steadily with an overall sense of peace and relaxation occurring throughout her body.[5] This clinical description, of course, does not begin to convey the wondrous pleasure of orgasm.

This basic blueprint of female orgasm is quite parallel to the male experience of single orgasm. Some women become aroused just in this way and have one single powerful orgasm. Some women are able to have two or more discrete orgasms within the same self-pleasuring or lovemaking session. Other women have what the Taoists referred to as "valley orgasms," where arousal is increased and pleasure is sustained between multiple orgasms. There is no right way to orgasm. As you become orgasmic and multi-orgasmic, your body will find its own pleasure pattern. These patterns will differ not only from woman to woman but also often from orgasm to orgasm for the same woman. Now let's look at ways to cultivate arousal and orgasms.

GETTING HOT AND BOTHERED

Before self-pleasuring many women find it extremely arousing to read erotic literature or to see sexual images. Contrary to popular belief, many women are just as aroused by these experiences as men are. However, much of the erotic material we get exposed to in our normal life is written by and for men and caters to men's particular sexual fantasies. These images can be arousing for women but often are not. Some women have felt offended or even traumatized by pornographic images and literature. Fortunately, there are now many sources of erotic literature and film specifically by and for women. (For a few suggestions see the Resources at the end of the book.)

Some women dislike explicit erotica and instead find novels with romantic content more arousing. Whatever it is that you find stimulating, from Harlequin to hard-core, there is absolutely nothing wrong with using them in your own self-cultivation. Fantasy is an integral part of our sexuality.

Some women's sexual imagination is so strong that they can experience orgasm simply from their own internal imagery without being touched. Beverly Whipple, Gina Ogden, and Barry Komisaruk measured these women's physical responses in a clinical setting and proved their ability to orgasm from fantasy alone.[6] Never underestimate the power of the mind. As you learn to channel your sexual energy throughout your body in chapter 3, you will learn to experience a wave of orgasmic pleasure throughout your body whenever you wish.

Some women feel guilty about their fantasies because they may involve content that is arousing but disturbing to them. For example, women may fantasize about experiences that they would never want to have happen in their real life, such as rape. There is no reason to be ashamed about what arouses you. As long as sex itself is safe and consensual, there need be no shame about it. Our sex life is a complex web of instinct, experience, and imagination. We could no more separate these strands than we could pull apart a spider's own intricate and delicate web. It is important to note that our fantasy life functions best when free of judgment or restraints. We must be responsible for our actions, but in our imagination we have complete freedom.

HANDY HELPERS

Many women find that they are much more easily aroused with the use of a vibrator or dildo during self-cultivation. There are a wide variety of vibrators and dildos on the market, and we suggest obtaining one from a store where you can find real help in getting one that you feel comfortable with. You can also obtain these through mail order or over the Internet if you prefer. (For listings, see Resources.) As with all sex toys, experiment to see which particular use arouses you most. Many women prefer a vibrator to stimulate the clitoris and a dildo for penetration. There are dildos in all sizes and shapes to suit individual preferences or for particular uses (such as G-spot stimulation). Some sex toys are designed for anal stimulation. The only way to know what works for you is to try it out. Some stores even permit buyers to test-drive (using safe sex precautions) at the store!

RELAXATION AND A SENSE OF HUMOR

The handmaiden of arousal and orgasm is relaxation.

The handmaiden of arousal and orgasm is relaxation. There are perhaps no greater enemies to sexual pleasure than anxiety and stress. When you begin to feel anxious, stop and take deep breaths as we learned in the Belly Breathing exercise on page 35.

Another great antidote to anxiety and fear is laughter. Keeping a sense of humor about exploring pleasure alone and with a partner will be an invaluable asset. We all feel a little silly and maybe not so sexy when we begin to explore our pleasure for the first time. "I can't believe I'm ___ years old, and I'm lying here with this battery-operated thingamajig trying to get myself off!" It's healthy to laugh about it. But then continue with your body exploration. It may take several sessions of self-pleasuring before you find the techniques that set you off. Remember that finding your pleasure points, regardless of whether or not you have an orgasm, will be a sweet reward.

As with the last exercise, set the stage for your self-pleasuring by being sure you will not be interrupted for at least thirty minutes. Do whatever it is that helps you relax: taking a bath, exercising, drinking a small glass of wine,[7] playing music, lighting candles, and so forth.

BUILDING TO ORGASM

1. PLEASURE YOURSELF: Using the techniques you learned in the last exercise, begin touching yourself, starting first with hands, feet, legs, and arms and moving in gradually to the more erogenous zones—nipples, clitoris, and vagina. As before, experiment with different kinds of strokes and different areas of stimulation.

2. TRY TEASING YOURSELF: There is no hurry here. When you feel yourself building toward orgasm, prolong the experience by touching places that are somewhat less sensitive and then returning to more sensitive spots. Bring yourself close to orgasm and then back off several times. By doing this you increase the intensity of the orgasm.

3. TRY A HANDY HELPER: If you are not easily or frequently orgasmic, it may take several sessions before you are able to have an orgasm with self-stimulation. If you are not successful with manual stimulation and you feel comfortable, try using a vibrator. As mentioned, many women find that using a vibrator for clitoral stimulation is the quickest and easiest way to orgasm.

4. AN ATTITUDE OF GRATITUDE: After an orgasm or after stopping the exercise, take some time to continue stroking your body. Be grateful to your body for providing so much pleasure. And most important, be grateful to yourself for taking the time to give yourself the gift of self-love.

Many women find that using a vibrator for clitoral stimulation is the quickest and easiest way to orgasm.

If you are not able to have an orgasm on the first several tries, be patient with yourself. Any amount of pleasure you experience is good in and of itself. Orgasm is not the ultimate goal; the ultimate goal is to find pleasure in your body. All that is necessary to practice self-cultivation and Taoist lovemaking is the arousal of sexual energy, or chi. For further information on difficulty with orgasm, read the section "Missing the Big Bang: Overcoming Anorgasmia" (anorgasmia is the absence of orgasm) at the end of this chapter. The following exercises for strengthening your PC muscle will also help you intensify the pleasure you already experience and help you on your way to multi-orgasmic lovemaking.

Your Sex Muscle

If you had to pick one muscle that is essential to your sexual pleasure and fulfillment, it would be your PC muscle, sometimes called your love muscle

Exercising this muscle is far more important to your sexual life than all the hours spent working out in the gym.

or sex muscle. Exercising this muscle is far more important to your sexual life than all the hours spent working out in the gym. Strengthening your pubococcygeus (or PC) muscle will help you have orgasms when you wish, improve you ability to have multiple orgasms, and give you the strength to pleasure your partner intensely during intercourse.

Your PC muscle is a muscular sling at the bottom of your pelvis that supports all of your sexual and reproductive organs as well as your urethra and rectum. Contracting your PC muscle will increase the pleasure you feel and the ease with which you can have orgasms from both clitoral and vaginal stimulation. Beverly Whipple, coauthor of *The G Spot*, explains, "The stronger the PC muscle . . . the greater a woman's orgasmic response." Strengthening your PC muscle "is the most important thing you can do to improve your chances of having multiple orgasms."[8] When you contract your PC muscle you improve the blood flow to the vagina and perineum, which increases your sexual energy and lubrication.

A woman's PC muscle, which is important for becoming multi-orgasmic, extends from the pubic bone to the tailbone.

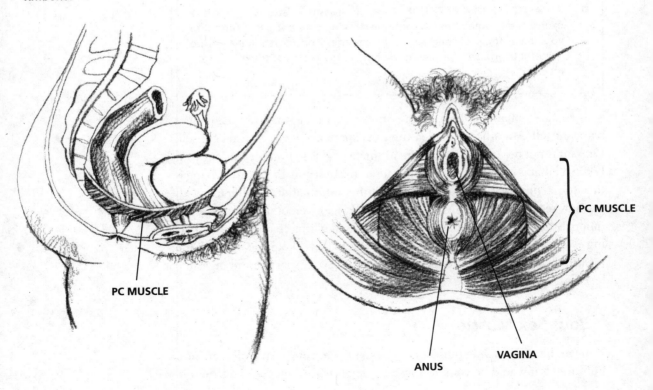

PC MUSCLE

PC MUSCLE

ANUS   VAGINA

You may have heard of the PC muscle in connection with childbirth. Physicians recommend that women do PC exercises called Kegels (pronounced KAY-gulls) prior to and after the birth of children.[9] Kegel exercises are designed to strengthen this muscle and improve its elasticity during the birth process. They also increase the muscular support of the vagina and uterus after birth and with aging.

As we grow older the strength of the PC muscle decreases unless it is regularly exercised. If a woman has had several vaginal births, the muscle is further weakened. This is why many women start to have difficulty holding in their urine in their fifties, sixties, and seventies. Strengthening this muscle is an important part of maintaining our general health as well as realizing our sexual potential.

As we grow older the strength of the PC muscle decreases unless it is regularly exercised.

STRENGTHENING YOUR PC MUSCLE

Learning how to contract your PC muscle can sometimes be a challenge. The next time you need to urinate, stop the urine stream and then start it again several times as you empty your bladder. It is your PC muscle that you are contracting in order to do this. The sensation should be that you are pulling your urethra and vaginal area up slightly into your body.

If you are not able to stop the stream of urine, your PC muscle is weak. Do not be concerned, for like any muscle in the body, your PC muscle can be strengthened with regular exercise. (If you find that you sometimes have difficulty holding in your urine, particularly when coughing, sneezing, or laughing, or you find that you just cannot make it to the toilet in time, there may be other anatomical problems that you should discuss with your physician. Kegel exercises are still highly recommended for this problem, but it would be wise to seek your physician's advice.)

Some women find themselves pushing down instead of pulling up when they initially start to do PC muscle strengthening. It is important that you become familiar enough with what it feels like to lift and squeeze your PC muscle. These exercises do not require that you use your abdominal muscles. In fact, the exercises work much better if the rest of your muscles are relaxed.

When first learning these exercises, it's very helpful to have something to contract your PC muscle against (e.g., a finger or a dildo). The resistance will allow you to squeeze with more strength.

Exercise 10

VAGINAL SQUEEZES

1. Lie down or sit down on the edge of a chair or on the toilet and insert two lubricated fingers into your vagina.

2. Squeeze your PC muscle around your fingers. You should feel a slight contraction of the walls of your vagina, approximately one inch from the entrance of your vagina.

3. Spread your fingers apart, as when making a peace sign. Contract the muscle again and see if you can bring your fingers together. If you cannot, your PC requires further strengthening.

Once you get the hang of how to contract your PC muscle, exercising it is fairly simple and easy to do. There are many different techniques for exercising the PC muscle with varying lengths of contraction and repetitions. A common recommendation is to contract the muscle and hold it for ten seconds and then release. If you are unable to hold it that long, hold it as long as you can and then release. You may want to start doing this ten times and work up to doing it fifty times three times a day.

Finding the Way

Ring Muscles

The traditional Taoist technique for exercising the PC muscle is extremely helpful. It uses the Taoist awareness that all circular muscles of the body (around the eyes, mouth, urethra, vagina, and anus) are connected. By squeezing the muscles around your eyes and mouth it is possible to increase the force of your PC exercises. Contracting the muscles around your eyes involves simply squinting, and contracting the muscles of your mouth involves simply sucking, like a baby nurses. It is also helpful to squeeze the PC muscle on exhalation, as it helps you relax the rest of your muscles and isolate the PC.

It may also be of use to do PC exercises against a dildo or your partner's penis. You may find that contracting your PC muscle during lovemaking increases your arousal remarkably. Contracting your PC muscle increases the sexual energy in your pelvic region and spreads a warm flush of arousal throughout your body. Contracting against a penis or dildo as it is withdrawn from your vagina can be extremely stimulating, as it creates suction against the vaginal walls. You may want to experiment with what feels best for you.

As your muscle gets stronger and stronger, your lover will certainly be able to appreciate the increased contractions against his penis during lovemaking. Most men find this extremely arousing. The Taoists strongly recommended that a woman squeeze around *the shaft* of the man's penis, which will invigorate his whole body (see chapter 5) and allow him to experience very high levels of pleasure without ejaculating. This technique can also prolong the amount of time you can make love and increase both of your chances to become multi-orgasmic.

Exercise 11

PC PULL-UPS

1. **INHALE AND CONCENTRATE:** Inhale and concentrate on your vagina.

2. **EXHALE AND CONTRACT:** As you exhale, contract your PC muscle.

3. **INHALE AND RELAX:** Inhale and relax your muscles.

4. **REPEAT—EXHALE/CONTRACT AND INHALE/RELAX:** Continue contracting your muscles as you exhale and releasing them as you inhale. Contract and release with your breathing, starting with eighteen times at first, and then working up to thirty-six times or more. (After each set of eighteen, rest before continuing.)

5. **CONTRACT AS LONG AS YOU CAN:** Now repeat the exercise, but this time on each exhalation contract your PC muscle as long as you can and then release. Do nine long contractions, and then rest before doing another set.

One of the results of doing PC muscle exercises is that they may arouse sexual energy in you no matter where you are. This can certainly add zing to a boring business meeting! If you can simply enjoy the warm energy, that is fine. However, some women find the increased sexual energy distracting. If this is the case for you, you will need to learn the exercises in chapter 3 that show you how to channel this energy up to the brain in order to increase your energy level and concentration.

Becoming Multi-Orgasmic

Women have the capacity for virtually inexhaustible sexual pleasure. Yet while all women have the capacity to have multiple orgasms, many do not experience them or do not experience them regularly. Why do some women have them while others do not? Why does the same woman have them sometimes and not other times? Certainly many women who didn't think that they could have multiple orgasms have discovered that they could as they have had new sexual experiences and new partners or have become more sexually experienced.

In Alfred Kinsey's famous studies of sexuality in the 1950s, only approximately 14 percent of women were multi-orgasmic. By 1970 the number of multi-orgasmic women had increased to only 16 percent.[10] And even today far fewer women are multi-orgasmic than one might expect. Contrary to popular belief, currently only 15 to 25 percent of women are multiply orgasmic.[11]

Recently an anonymous questionnaire was sent out to 805 college-educated female nurses, which showed that a surprising 43 percent of the respondents had experienced multiple orgasms.[12] So how did these women get so lucky?

Contrary to popular belief, currently only 15 to 25 percent of women are multiply orgasmic.

WHAT DO MULTI-ORGASMIC WOMEN DO DIFFERENTLY?

This same study took an in-depth look at what characteristics differentiate those women who are multi-orgasmic from those who are singly orgasmic.

Self-Pleasure: Multi-orgasmic women are more likely to masturbate and to have been orgasmic at an earlier age. While this could be attributed to some greater innate sexual drive, it is more likely that these women grew up in an environment that was more open to sexual exploration or were simply lucky enough to stumble on orgasms early in their life. One multi-orgasmic woman we interviewed for this book developed a great fondness for the bathtub faucet as a child after her first orgasmic experience there. She never refused taking a bath after that.

These early experiences of orgasm condition our body to become accustomed to having orgasms. Though we can't go back and change our childhood experiences, we certainly can now begin having more orgasms, which will condition our body to do so again and again. The body works by habit. We don't think a whole lot about driving when we're behind the wheel of a car or about brushing our teeth when we're getting ready for bed. Any patterned behavior is the same. With experience we develop habitual neural pathways by which our body knows how to operate. Orgasm is no different. The more you have it, the more you *can* have it.

Know Their Pleasure Spots: Multi-orgasmic women are more sexually explorative. This doesn't mean that multi-orgasmic women need to be interested in sex toys or bondage. It simply means that they have explored (or allowed their partner to explore) their sexual landscape. They know the places on their body that make them swoon and that make them sing. As you do the exercises in this book and discover your pleasure points, you will know how to pleasure yourself and how to help your partner pleasure you.

Stimulate Themselves Physically and Mentally: Multi-orgasmic women stimulate their clitoris during sex or have their partner do so. Since the clitoris is the key sexual organ for most women it is absolutely vital that we stimulate it ourselves or have our partner stimulate it when we are trying to orgasm.

Multi-orgasmic women are also more likely to use vaginal stimulation when masturbating and more likely to orgasm with vaginal penetration from their partner. Not only do they optimize clitoral stimulation; they optimize stimulation of their sensitive vaginal spots.

They also more often seek and receive nipple stimulation and keep their mind stimulated by using sexual fantasies, erotic film, and literature.

Ask for What They Want: Multi-orgasmic women are able to ask for what they want or direct their partner's hands, mouth, or penis to where they want it. They are more likely to give and receive oral sex. They also stimulate or have their partner stimulate a variety of erogenous zones at the same time. They mix and match their stimulation, joining nipple stimulation with clitoral stimulation, clitoral stimulation with deep vaginal or G-spot stimulation.

It is not a mystery why these women are able to have multiple orgasms. They stimulate all of their most sensitive areas more frequently and have partners who are willing to do the same.

So what about you? Using tips from these multi-orgasmic women and the skills you have already learned, the following nine steps will help you have multiple orgasms whenever you want them. If you want to have multiple orgasms with your partner, it is a good idea to encourage him (or her) to read this short nine-step program. Your partner will be a much more able assistant if he has read these few pages.

With experience we develop habitual neural pathways by which our body knows how to operate. Orgasm is no different. The more you have it, the more you *can* have it.

Nine Steps to Multiple Orgasms for Any Woman

STEP 1: YOU MUST BELIEVE

Orgasms do not happen between the legs; they happen between the ears. We know that this is true because even people who are paraplegic or quadriplegic and have no sensation below their belt still experience orgasm with stimulation of other parts of their body (for example, their chest or neck). Many women who think that they are unable to have multiple orgasms discover that this is not the case when they "accidentally" have a second orgasm. You have to believe that you can have more than one orgasm and consciously work toward it. Though it may take persistence to experience multiple orgasms the first time, remember that the more you do it, the easier and faster you will have them the next time.

Orgasms do not happen between the legs; they happen between the ears.

STEP 2: TURN ON YOUR MIND

A woman's imagination is the primary instrument of her desire, so don't forget to use it. Remember that the more aroused you feel, the more sexual energy you have and the easier it will be to have multiple orgasms.

We explored what arouses you in the early part of the chapter. Don't forget to use this self-knowledge now. You can anticipate lovemaking with fleeting sexual touches or prolonged kisses during the day. You can also arrange the setting with lighting and scents that stimulate your sensual mind. If certain locations or times of day feel more erotic to you, then do it there and then. Sometimes a surprise afternoon appointment with your lover can be much more satisfying than sleepy bedtime sex.

If you like, explore erotic literature or film. Sharing these with your partner could be an enjoyable prelude to lovemaking. The stronger your fantasy life, the easier it will be to increase your arousal when you wish.

While fantasy is an important part of self-cultivation and lovemaking, fantasizing about someone other than your partner while making love *with* your partner can distract you from the exchange of energy taking place between you. Taoist lovemaking exemplifies the subtle blending of each other's sexual energies in order to renew each other's physical and spiritual strength. If you are not mentally present with your partner, this energetic exchange cannot take place. This doesn't mean, however, that you can't fantasize at all during lovemaking, only that you need to be emotionally and spiritually present with your partner. For example, you could imagine that the two of you are alone on a warm Caribbean beach instead of in your bedroom in Baltimore.

STEP 3: STIMULATE MULTIPLE PLEASURE POINTS

Multi-orgasmic women enhance their arousal by stimulating multiple pleasure points. Some of these (clitoris, G spot) are so important that they will be discussed in detail below. You will have discovered your own hot spots in the body exploration at the beginning of the chapter.

If touching the curve of your ear makes you crazy or caressing the insides of your wrists makes you writhe, stroke these during self-pleasuring or let your lover in on the secret. Sucking on fingers or toes is a wonderful foreshadowing of more intense stimulation to come.

Many women find nipple stimulation extremely arousing. In fact, some women can orgasm from nipple stimulation alone. If you are someone who enjoys nipple play, it can be a tremendous source for increasing sexual energy. You can stimulate your own nipples during self-pleasuring or partnered sex. Most partners will find it highly erotic to watch you stimulating yourself.

Women differ greatly from one another in the sensitivity of their nipples and how they like to be touched. Some women always prefer a featherlight touch. Other women find rougher handling of their breasts and nipples, including nipple squeezing and pulling, hard sucking, and rolling of the nipples, to be very erotic. In general, most women prefer lighter touches when they are less aroused and more intense touching when they are more aroused.

Sometimes having your nipples stimulated at the wrong time or in the wrong way can cause pain or nausea. It is important to demonstrate to your partner how you like to be touched and to give continual feedback—verbal or nonverbal—about what you like. If you are someone who does not have particularly sensitive nipples, keep in mind that, like any other part of your body, the more focused attention your breasts receive, the more sensitive they will become.

Remember that all bodily titillation will raise your *ching*, or sexual energy, and make it easier to crest over into second, third, and even fourth orgasms.

STEP 4: FOLLOW THE WAY OF THE TONGUE

If vibrators are perhaps the easiest way for women to have orgasms during self-pleasuring, oral sex is probably the easiest way for women to have orgasms during sex with their partner. It's hard to surpass the intense pleasure of direct clitoral stimulation with the soft malleable surface of the tongue and the sucking of the mouth. In the 1950s oral sex was considered taboo in the United States, but since the sexual revolution in the 1960s and 1970s, oral sex has become widely accepted and frequently practiced.

Multi-orgasmic women enhance their arousal by stimulating multiple pleasure points.

If vibrators are perhaps the easiest way for women to have orgasms during self-pleasuring, oral sex is probably the easiest way for women to have orgasms during sex with their partner.

When Susan Crain Bakos interviewed multi-orgasmic women for her book *Sexual Pleasures*, she found that those women who did experience multiple orgasms typically had the first orgasm while receiving oral sex. They reported that they could more easily experience another orgasm after oral sex than they could if their first orgasm had occurred during intercourse or manual stimulation. "Their other 'secret' was varied stimulation; cunnilingus often followed by intercourse with simultaneous manual stimulation. Also, they frequently made subtle shifts in position to get the sensations where and how they wanted them."[13] The tongue is a perfect instrument for stimulating the clitoris because it is strong, flexible, and soft.

Many more couples regularly practice cunnilingus now than they did forty years ago, but there are still couples who for various reasons do not make cunnilingus an active part of their sex life.

Discomfort with cunnilingus may be on the part of the giver or the receiver. Surprisingly, we find that most of the time women themselves are more uncomfortable with the idea of oral sex than are their partners.

The major reason for this discomfort seems to be concern about having one's mouth or one's partner's mouth near the genital and excretory area. (In other words, "It's dirty down there.") It might be enlightening to know that the variety and concentration of bacteria in one's mouth easily rivals the concentration of bacteria on the perineum or vaginal areas. One is not going to "get dirty" by kissing one's lover's genitals. If you bathe regularly, your genitals are certainly clean enough for your lover to kiss.

The vagina cleans itself quite satisfactorily. Putting any other substances in it to "freshen" it only disturbs its healthy balance. We would not recommend douching at any time, unless recommended by your doctor, as it disturbs the healthy bacteria that live in your vagina.

You should avoid using soap on the genital area as the various additives and perfumes in soaps can be irritating to the sensitive skin of the vagina and genital area. Washing off with water as part of general bathing (and before oral sex if you'd like) is usually sufficient. Using a cup of water to wash off while sitting on the toilet or in the bath or shower is quick and easy. (Detachable showerheads are also helpful, but watch out for the shower massage—you may not get out!)

Each woman's vaginal secretions have their own unique scent. This scent changes throughout the month with hormonal fluctuations and can even be affected by what you eat. For most men the smell of a woman's genitals is pleasant and for many even a turn-on. There are biological and evolutionary reasons why this is the case. If your partner is "*scent*-ually stunted" or is turned off by your scent, try bathing together, and as a last resort you can substitute finger play for tongue play.

The only time that a woman's vagina has an unpleasant smell is if she has an infection. If you note that you have increasing discharge and/or foul odor, you should consult your doctor.

If your partner has not yet become a cunnilingus connoisseur, refer him to the couples chapter. For most men, it is not the idea or even the smell that keeps them from becoming adept at cunnilingus but the fear that they won't know what they're doing. You can be of great help in pointing out what feels good and showing your partner where you're sensitive. A little positive reinforcement can work wonders.

STEP 5: TEASE YOURSELF

The following method of teasing is a classic sexual technique that every woman should have in her sexual repertoire. It can greatly enhance sexual pleasure and increase the likelihood of orgasm and multiple orgasms. The technique is simple but very effective.

Arouse yourself or have your partner arouse you to a point of low to moderate desire, and then back off on the stimulation you are receiving so that your desire decreases somewhat but does not disappear completely. Then increase stimulation again so that your desire increases to above the level that it was at previously. Now back off slightly on stimulation again. Continue slowly increasing the level of your arousal and backing off slightly prior to orgasm. This will increase the intensity of your pleasure, and, when you do orgasm, your sexual energy will be very high. Immediately following orgasm, begin stimulation again to maintain your level of arousal. Using the stimulation and backing-off technique will allow you to build to another orgasm.

Some women find that their sensitive spots, be they vaginal, clitoral, nipple, or whatever, are hypersensitive at the time of orgasm or just after. If this is the case for you, have your lover stop stimulation for a short period of time (less than thirty seconds) but then continue to stimulate you. If you wait too long to restart stimulation after the first orgasm, your body may move into a refractory period, making a second orgasm less likely.

While this method of teasing can stoke your sexual fire, being teased for too long can be frustrating. If you are practicing this with your partner, be sure to communicate when your erotic suspense is turning to boredom and you want to move on to the next step.

STEP 6: GO, SPOT, GO

Earlier in the chapter we discussed the location of the G spot. In addition to this famous spot, you may also have found other "spots" of your own. Remember that these sensitive spots are better found when you are fully aroused. Many women report having found their G spot accidentally, sometimes after decades of intercourse with the same partner. It is more than worth your time to try different angles of penetration with fingers, penis, or dildo to see if you have any particularly sensitive areas of your vagina. Having vaginal in addition to clitoral stimulation greatly enhances the pleasure and likelihood of having multiple orgasms.

Many women find that their first orgasms come primarily from their clitoris while their later orgasms, when they're more fully aroused, occur more deeply in their vagina. These deeper orgasms can be extremely satisfying. Since different nerves carry the sensations from the vagina and the clitoris to the brain, some authors have suggested that vaginal orgasms are quite different from clitoral orgasms. The clitoral orgasm is more akin to the penile orgasm, with clitoral engorgement and repetitive contractions of the PC muscle. With the vaginal orgasm, the woman begins to have deeper contractions and pleasure spreading throughout the pelvis.

The Brauers studied women capable of having these deep vaginal orgasms and recorded their EEGs (which monitor brain waves). These tracings showed that women in the throes of deep vaginal orgasms have the same brain wave patterns as people who are in deep meditation."[14]

These deep vaginal orgasms were well known to women in China who practiced the Tao. The Taoist egg exercises that have been used for centuries to strengthen a woman's vagina can enhance the experience of these orgasms (see the woman's chapter in *The Multi-Orgasmic Man*, "Satisfaction Guaranteed"). The sexual energy created by these orgasms can easily be circulated throughout the body to create whole-body orgasms, as will be discussed in chapter 3. The Taoists also believed these deep vaginal orgasms are extremely healing and could energize the rest of the body. We will discuss this more in chapter 5.

During intercourse, one of the best positions for stimulating the G spot is to have the man enter the woman from behind, while the woman is on hands and knees or lying down flat on her stomach (see illustration opposite). This allows the man to move up over her in a more vertical position and to use slightly shallower thrusting to stimulate her G spot. The G spot usually lies

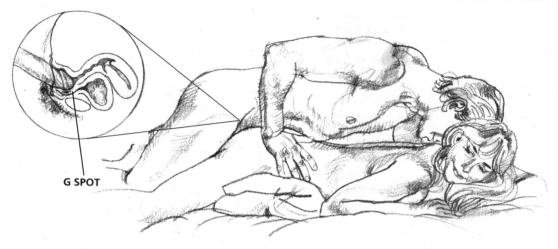

G SPOT

only a few inches inside her vagina through the anterior (front) wall of her vagina (see illustration on p. 32). Another variation is to have the man on his back and the woman on top facing the man's feet. Still another variation is for the woman, when on top facing the man's feet, to recline back on her hands toward her partner's chest. In any of these positions, she can control the depth of penetration and guide his penis to stimulate her G spot. Whatever method works best for you to stimulate your G spot, this orgasmic trigger point is sure to help you double, triple, or quadruple your pleasure.

STEP 7: USE YOUR PC MUSCLE

In the section on strengthening your PC muscle, we discussed at length the importance of this muscle to orgasmic potential. Contracting the PC muscle is one of the primary methods the Taoist sexual experts used to get sexual energy flowing in the body. When practicing the PC exercises, you may also have noticed that it increases your desire. When you contract your PC muscle during lovemaking it has the same effect, increasing your pleasure and moving you closer to multiple orgasms.

As your sexual energy rises with PC muscle contractions, your heart rate will increase and your breathing will shorten. Stimulating your clitoris or hitting a sensitive vaginal spot at this time will often push you over into orgasm. Since it is the PC muscle that contracts with orgasm, having a strong PC muscle will also make the pleasurable rhythmic contractions of orgasm more intense.

The G spot can be stimulated when the man is behind and the woman lies on her belly. A pillow under her waist can sometimes help. Detail shows how the angle of the penis in this position stimulates the G spot.

Finding the Way

PC Secrets

Here are several PC techniques to try that will pleasure you and your partner:

- STIMULATING THE ENTRANCE: When your partner (or dildo) enters you, contract rhythmically around the head of his penis to stimulate the entrance to the vagina.

- SUCKING YOUR PARTNER IN: Have your partner slowly penetrate you while you rhythmically contract your PC as if you were sucking your partner into your vagina.

- SQUEEZING DURING WITHDRAWAL: With regular in-and-out thrusting, squeeze your PC while your partner withdraws. This creates suction against your vaginal walls, which can be quite pleasurable.

- STAYING DEEP INSIDE: When your partner is deep inside you, have him remain still while you contract your PC muscle against him.

- CONTRACTING SHORT AND LONG: Using the traditional Taoist thrusting technique of nine shallow and one deep (see chapter 4), squeeze briefly as your partner withdraws during the shallow thrusts. During the long deep thrust, squeeze continuously as he slides in and out.

Like any exercise, these PC techniques can be difficult or tiring at first. Start slowly and do what is comfortable and pleasurable. With time, your increased strength and control of your PC muscle will add greatly to your orgasmic ability and your partner's pleasure.

STEP 8: STIMULATE THE CLITORIS AND VAGINA TOGETHER

Whether you are self-pleasuring or making love with your partner, make sure you optimize clitoral touch. In particular, a great many women require clitoral stimulation with intercourse in order to orgasm. As sex researchers Alan P. Brauer and Donna J. Brauer note, "When a man's penis is thrusting in a woman's vagina, he's directly stimulating his most sensitive organ [the head of his penis], but only indirectly stimulating hers."[15] There are various ways to stimulate your clitoris during intercourse. Your partner can use his hands, which is easier in certain positions, such as woman on top or "doggie style," with the man behind.

Some women find it extremely pleasurable to have their clitoris rubbed by their partner's pubis during intercourse. This is easiest with you on top in a kneeling position so that you can direct the amount of pressure you want. This can also be done with the man on top if he places his pubis against his partner's clitoris. You can experiment with different positions to find which works best for you.

It is also more than okay to stimulate your own clitoris during intercourse. Most lovers find it *highly* erotic to see their partner stimulating herself to orgasm. If your partner feels left out, he can rest his fingers on yours or you can rest yours on his.

If it's your vibrator that really gets you going, there's no reason that you can't use it during intercourse. The vibrations might also stimulate your partner. If your partner feels territorial about having the only "long, hard thing" in the bedroom, you may want to explain that he is not being replaced, just complemented. Explain that since you have multiple pleasurable spots, it helps you to have more than one of them stimulated at the same time. You can also give him a turn stimulating you with the vibrator before or during lovemaking.

STEP 9: ASK FOR A HELPING HAND

If you're trying to experience multiple orgasms with self-pleasuring, this step does not apply since you can follow your own whims. However, most women who want to experience multiple orgasms also want to do so with a partner.

Asking your partner for what you need and want is vital to your ability to have multiple orgasms. It is worth remembering that the success of your sexual communication is dependent on your overall ability to communicate openly with your partner. What goes on in the bedroom (or wherever you happen to make love) is not separate from the rest of your life together. If you feel anger or resentment toward your partner, it will carry over into your sexual relationship. Try to resolve negative feelings before sexual exploration. (Please see chapter 6, "Making Real Love," for a longer discussion of emotional and sexual intimacy.)

Your partner must also be interested and invested in your having multiple orgasms. Your lover needs to be willing to try different positions and types of stimulation and to listen to your directions (verbal and nonverbal) about what you need. If you sense some reluctance in your partner, remind him that the energy he invests will result in great rewards for your sex life as well as a much happier, more satisfied you!

On the other hand, some men are so *personally* invested in their partner having an orgasm (or many) that they see it as a lack of their own abilities if she does not. Although this attitude may be an improvement over the grunt-and-roll-over phenomenon, having a partner who is obsessed with your having multiple orgasms will not help you to do so. You must be in a playful and relaxed mood to have a second orgasm, which is difficult when the goal of multiple orgasms becomes all-important.

The pressure of having to have multiple orgasms to please *him* can prevent you from having multiple orgasms that please *you*. Remind him that your body is *your* body and your level of pleasure is not a reflection of his skill as a lover, your attraction to him, or your affection for him. Explain that, unlike chocolate and flowers, an orgasm cannot be given to you. You need to allow yourself to have an orgasm. Or to put it into guy language, you need to be the *quarterback*, and you need to call the plays.

From your experiences in self-touching and finding your sensitive spots, you should now have a good idea of how you like to be touched and stimulated. It is vital that you be able to communicate this to your partner during lovemaking. Most partners appreciate feedback about how they're doing. Remember that it can be frustrating for your partner to try to please you if he does not hear what you like or dislike.

Giving good feedback is a loving art. The bedroom is a vulnerable place, where we are naked both physically and emotionally. Be careful to focus on

> The pressure of having to have multiple orgasms to please *him* can prevent you from having multiple orgasms that please *you*.

telling your partner what you like and what you want rather than on what you don't like.

For example, it is not usually as successful to say, "Stop that!" or "That hurts!" or "You're not doing it right!" The result is usually withdrawal and hurt feelings. If your partner is trying to please you, it is important not to be judgmental of his attempts. Criticism will dampen your partner's sexual desire as well as his or her desire to please you. If you don't like what your partner is doing, it is much more effective to say, "Try it a little more over here," or "A little lighter pressure. Yeah, that's good." As in any learning process, lots of positive feedback is always helpful.

If it is difficult to talk to your partner during lovemaking, or if it breaks your concentration on your pleasure, use nonverbal sounds and talk about it later. But don't forget to talk about it. As embarrassing as it might seem at first, it is essential to the strengthening of your sexual relationship (not to mention your relationship in general).

Whether or not you feel comfortable telling your partner what you want, don't forget the power of nonverbal sounds to direct your partner to the places and ways you'd like to be touched. Be generous with your moans, ooohs, and aaahhhs. Not only do they encourage the kind of touch you want; they turn your partner on, too. Most men consider their partner's satisfied sounds to be the greatest aphrodisiac.

Try out each of the nine steps alone or with a partner, then adapt them to suit your own rhythm and sexual tastes. The following exercise distills the nine steps into a helpful sequence for easy reference. All women have different preferences. You should explore any combination of the nine steps that works for you.

Finally, do not worry if you do not have multiple orgasms on the first try. Try to see your attempts to reach multiple orgasms as a playful, exploratory process that gives you great sensual rewards all along the way. Taoist sexuality is about increasing your pleasure and sexual energy and about harmonizing with your partner, which you do when you experience pleasure, whether or not you have an orgasm. While orgasms are wonderful, they are just peaks within a mountain range of pleasure.

Giving good feedback is a loving art. The bedroom is a vulnerable place, where we are naked both physically and emotionally.

Most men consider their partner's satisfied sounds to be the greatest aphrodisiac.

Exercise 12

BECOMING A MULTI-ORGASMIC WOMAN

1. YOU MUST BELIEVE: You can have multiple orgasms. Choose a date and time for your multi-orgasmic play, and keep it!

2. TURN ON YOUR MIND: Create a sensual atmosphere for lovemaking and use your imagination or erotic literature/film to explore your fantasy life.

3. STIMULATE MULTIPLE PLEASURE POINTS: Start with full-body caresses and move toward your hot spots: neck, ears, nipples.

4. FOLLOW THE WAY OF THE TONGUE: If with a partner, begin with cunnilingus. If by yourself, use a vibrator for stimulating your clitoris. Also continue stimulating your other pleasure points.

5. TEASE YOURSELF: With cunnilingus or with a vibrator, use the teasing technique of stimulating and backing off. Then have your first orgasm. Restart pleasuring yourself within thirty seconds.

6. GO, SPOT, GO: Move slowly to penetration. If with your partner, use positions that stimulate the G spot (for example, man from behind with the woman lying on her stomach). If by yourself, use a vibrator or dildo to stimulate your G spot.

7. USE YOUR PC MUSCLE: Contract around your partner's penis or your vibrator or dildo, using whichever PC muscle technique feels good to you.

8. STIMULATE THE CLITORIS AND VAGINA TOGETHER: Continue to stimulate your clitoris during penetration.

9. ASK FOR A HELPING HAND: Tell your partner what feels good and what you need. Now ride your pleasure to another wave of orgasm. Congratulations! You are a multi-orgasmic woman.

Missing the Big Bang: Overcoming Anorgasmia

While Taoist sexuality is not nearly as goal oriented as our Western view of sex, it does appreciate the importance of orgasm for both our pleasure and our health. This section is for those women who are having difficulty experiencing the regular sexual pleasure that they want even after completing the exercises earlier in the chapter.

Our sexual desire waxes and wanes according to our overall health and the events in our life. However, women who have never been able to orgasm, either by self-stimulation or with a partner, are considered to be "anorgas-mic," or "without orgasm." The good news is that at least 90 percent of women who have never had an orgasm will be able to experience one.

Practicing self-stimulation and learning where you are most sensitive is the key to becoming orgasmic. All sex experts on anorgasmia recommend doing exercises as described at the beginning of the chapter to explore and stimu-late your body. You should do these exercises in a relaxed way for at least a week before going on to try to stimulate yourself to orgasm. For some women, just the chance to explore their body without the pressure of having to orgasm allows them to relax and increase their sexual energy to the point that they can orgasm when they do try.

Don't forget about the importance of increasing your desire in a relaxed, sensual atmosphere. Consider using music, candlelight, erotica, movies, or literature as you feel comfortable. If after several weeks you are still unable to orgasm, consider buying a vibrator. The majority of women orgasm most eas-ily with stimulation of their clitoris with a vibrator. (Consult the Resources at the end of the book for a store or Internet site to help you choose a vibrator that suits you.) However, you can certainly try to stimulate other vaginal spots, as discussed previously, as well. Try other means of stimulation also, such as the showerhead or a hot tub jet.

For many women it is the inability to relax their body and/or distracting repetitive thoughts in their mind that keeps them from experiencing orgasm. Orgasm requires letting go of rational thought and letting your body move as it wishes without your conscious control. This release of control is difficult for many people in our society. The belly breathing technique that we learned ear-lier in the chapter (Exercise 7) is essential for relaxing your mind and body.

You should use the belly breathing technique whenever you begin to feel anxious or tense during your self-stimulation exercises. It will also help quiet nagging thoughts in your mind that distract you from your bodily pleasure.

SHARING YOUR ORGASMS WITH YOUR PARTNER

Most sex therapists recommend using self-stimulation techniques until you can reliably have an orgasm by yourself. After experiencing orgasms by yourself, next you will no doubt want to have them with your partner. Most therapists recommend that, rather than hoping to have an orgasm during intercourse, you pleasure yourself to orgasm in front of your partner. This can be scary and embarrassing but is a wonderful way to show your partner what you like. Often this may feel more comfortable if your partner is willing to pleasure himself in front of you, too. This allows you to learn the techniques that he uses.

The next step is to do gentle touching with your partner without trying to orgasm. This can include sensual massage and sexual stimulation, the only requirement being that you remain relaxed and enjoy the experience. After a week or two of this nonpressured pleasure, have your partner pleasure you as you have been pleasing yourself all the way to orgasm.

All of these exercises require open and honest communication. If you have difficulty trusting your partner or cannot communicate about your pleasure, it will be difficult to experience orgasm together.

Since most women orgasm with their partner from stimulation other than intercourse, intercourse should be avoided until you are regularly able to orgasm while being touched in other ways. Remember, as we have said above, that using your fingers to stimulate yourself during intercourse is an excellent way to have an orgasm with your partner.

If you are still unable to orgasm there are many good places to find help. The book *Becoming Orgasmic* is a great place to begin (see Resources). We would also strongly encourage you to seek counseling from a sex therapist. Often there are early life experiences that can keep us from our full pleasure. Do not be afraid of exploring what may have been negative experiences with sexuality as a child or young person. Uncovering these may be the door to your sexual freedom.

Finally, there are physiologic influences on women's ability to become orgasmic. These will be discussed in more detail in the next section. Do not give up hope! With time and persistence almost all women are able to experience orgasm, and absolutely every woman can expand the pleasure she experiences during self-pleasuring and lovemaking.

Today we tend to see the mighty "O" as the be-all and end-all of sex. According to the Taoists, sex and the cultivation of sexual energy have a much broader and more important role as the basis of our vitality and health as well as our emotional and spiritual life. You can cultivate your sexual energy, feel great pleasure, improve your health, and expand the emotional and spiritual intimacy in your relationship even without having orgasms. In short, while we spend a great deal of time teaching men and women how to multiply their orgasms, orgasms are simply part of the larger process of expanding your sexual, creative, and energetic potential.

SITUATIONAL ANORGASMIA

Women who previously have been orgasmic and for whatever reason have stopped being able to experience orgasms are considered to have "situational" anorgasmia. Joy Davidson, an expert on what she calls "orgasmic disruption," says, "Women's orgasmic patterns are far more delicate than men's. . . . Men are often able to have an orgasm via physical stimulation alone while we tend to weave a tangled web of thought, physical potential, fantasy and emotion into each sexual encounter."[16]

If a woman has a new partner, increased stress at work or in the family, a change in medications, or a new home or phase of life, she may have a change in her orgasmic pattern. Usually this is attributable to one of several common causes.

PERIMENOPAUSE AND MENOPAUSE

Women who are entering perimenopause, from ages forty to fifty-five, often are experiencing some new and sudden fluctuations in their hormonal balance. In addition to dropping estrogen levels, which decrease lubrication of the vaginal area and can decrease desire, a woman also experiences a drop-off in her testosterone level. Testosterone appears to be one of the primary factors in women's libido and orgasmic potential. (For a longer discussion of the changes that take place around menopause, see "Sexual Health for Older Women" in chapter 8.)

Women who begin hormone replacement therapy at the time of menopause seem to have some increase in their sexual drive and sexual function. However, for most women, this is still not equivalent to the strength of their libido in their thirties and forties. Supplementing with testosterone has profoundly positive effects on sex drive. However, testosterone supplementation is still experimental, and its safety and potential side effects are not completely understood. If you are in this life stage and find your sex drive or orgasmic ability diminished, you may want to consult your physician about testosterone and other new therapies that are becoming available.

PREGNANCY AND POSTPARTUM

Women who are pregnant, postpartum, or breast-feeding also complain about loss of desire or sexual sensitivity. Though some women have significantly increased libido while pregnant, other women suffer a decrease in libido. In the postpartum period and when breast-feeding, almost all women have a decrease in sex drive as a result of the hormone prolactin, which is responsible for producing milk. Though this may be inconvenient for you (and your partner) for a period of time, your desire should soon return to normal once you are finished breast-feeding.

It should go without saying that breast-feeding is extremely important for the health of the growing baby and well worth the temporary dampening of sexual drive. Though your drive to initiate sex is often decreased, you may find that once you are actually being sexual with your partner, your pleasure and orgasmic potential are not diminished. Most new parents find they have precious little time to think about sex, let alone to do it. During this time, massage and continuing to touch your partner are essential for your physical as well as emotional well-being. (We discuss the important hormonal benefits of touch in chapter 4.) As breast-feeding decreases *and* the baby sleeps better (at last!), your desire will begin to return.

BIRTH CONTROL

Another common enemy of sex drive and orgasm is the birth control pill. Although some women actually experience an increase in sex drive on the birth control pill, most women have a decrease in their general libido and sexual responsiveness. The high estrogen and progesterone levels in the pill can often outweigh your natural testosterone levels. Oral contraceptives are an extremely effective form of birth control (possibly in part because many women who are on them don't want to have sex!).

If you need dependable birth control and are still planning to have children in the future, we would not recommend that you go off the pill. However, if the effect on your libido is extreme, you might want to consider alternative forms of contraception. Keep in mind that progesterone-only forms of birth control such as Depo-Provera (the shot taken every three months) and Norplant (the capsules inserted into your inner arm that last for six years) can have the same effect of decreasing libido. Other birth control methods that do not decrease sex drive unfortunately are more inconvenient and less reliable (condoms plus spermicide, diaphragm, cervical cap). One exception to this is the IUD, which both is extremely effective and has no hormonal effect on you.[17] The modern IUDs are extremely safe, but they are recommended only for women who have already conceived or given birth and are monogamous.[18]

ILLNESS AND MEDICATIONS

Any chronic illness can decrease sex drive and the ability to orgasm. In particular, diabetes, heart disease, and stroke can impair the physiologic process of orgasm. Severe or long-standing high blood pressure and high cholesterol can also have adverse effects, as can certain neurologic conditions.

Some of these effects can be reversed and/or treated with medications, so consult your physician for assistance.

Many medications can influence your sex drive as well. See the box below for a comprehensive list of the most frequently used. Some common offenders are antidepressants and antihypertensive medications. It would be worth discussing with your doctor whether there are other medications if the ones you are on seem to be negatively influencing your sex drive. Most physicians will not bring up this subject unless the patient specifically asks, so don't be shy. In many cases there are alternative medications available. In a few cases, the only optimal medication is one that will negatively influence your sex drive. Try to do everything else you can to optimize your sensual and sexual life if this is the case.

COMMON DRUGS THAT DECREASE YOUR LIBIDO

Amiodarone (Cordarone)	Methyldopa (Aldomet)
Amitriptyline (Elavil)	Metoclopramide (Reglan)
Carbamazepine (Tegretol)	Metoprolol (Lopressor)
Cimetidine (Tagamet)	Phenytoin (Dilantin)
Diazepam (Valium)	Progesterone
Digoxin (Lanoxin)	Propranolol (Inderal)
Ketoconazole (Nizoral)	Ranitidine (Zantac)
Lithium	Spironolactone (Aldactone)

COMMON DRUGS THAT DECREASE YOUR ABILITY TO ORGASM

Alcohol	Fluoxetine (Prozac)
Alprazolam (Xanax)	Labetolol (Trandate, Normodyne)
Amitriptyline (Elavil)	Methyldopa (Aldomet)
Amphetamines	Narcotics
Clonidine (Catapres)	Sertraline (Zoloft)
Diazepam (Valium)	

Recreational drugs can also have negative effects on your sexual functioning. Common offenders are cigarettes, alcohol, marijuana, opiates (heroin and others), speed, and hallucinogens. The best sex (and the best sexual energy) depends on a clean body, mind, and heart. Healing Love can be a more intense and healthier high than any artificial drug—with no hangover the next morning.

RELATIONSHIP AND LIFESTYLE

If there is no physiologic reason for your loss of orgasm, look at your relationship and lifestyle. Do you have a new partner? Are there emotional issues with a current partner? Is there open communication in your relationship? Is your partner caressing you enough? Are you getting the stimulation of your erogenous zones (clitoris, breasts, most sensitive vaginal areas) that you need?

Sexual satisfaction also depends on a lifestyle that supports the health of your body, mind, and spirit. Have circumstances in your life changed that have led to increased anxiety or decreased sleep? In order to have a healthy sex life, you have to have a healthy life. You need to be getting enough rest and have relaxed time to be sexual. If you don't already have one, you might consider starting an exercise program. Studies show that women who get thirty minutes of aerobic exercise three times a week reported an increased ability to climax after starting their exercise program. This may be the result of improved cardiovascular health, increased blood flow to the genital area, or just feeling more comfortable in and better about their body.[19]

Remember that if you have previously been able to experience orgasm, the likelihood of your being able to do so again is extremely high. Be patient. Do some of the exploratory exercises at the beginning of the chapter. If you are still having difficulty, you might want to consider consulting a sex therapist. In addition, one of the major signs of depression is decreased libido. If you feel that this might be the cause of your sexual difficulties, it is all the more important to consult a therapist or your physician.

Finally, as we discussed above, the Healing Love practice involves much more than orgasms. In the following chapters, as you open yourself up to greater pleasure, healing, intimacy, and spiritual growth, you will find sources of joy that make the question of whether you did or did not have an orgasm seem insignificant.

CHAPTER 3

Better than Chocolate, Better than Coffee: Expanding Your Orgasms and Your Energy

In this chapter, you will discover:

- How to Cultivate and Channel Your Sexual Energy
- How to Use Your Sexual Energy to Revitalize Yourself
- How to Have Whole-Body Orgasms

Multiplying your orgasms is marvelous, but it is really only the beginning. As you learn to cultivate your sexual energy, you can expand your orgasms throughout your body and generate sexual energy that will invigorate and heal you for hours after lovemaking. The Taoists recognized several levels of orgasm, each with ever greater levels of intensity and healing.

The Taoists recognized several levels of orgasm, each with ever greater levels of intensity and healing.

Finding the Way

Expanding Levels of Orgasm

- GENITAL ORGASM: The genital orgasm is the orgasm most often experienced. Genital orgasms are generally quick and do not release a great deal of healing energy.

- WHOLE-BODY ORGASM: The whole-body orgasm, which we describe in this chapter, comes from circulating the sexual energy to your brain and throughout your body.

- SOUL ORGASM: Finally, the soul orgasm, which we will discuss in chapter 7 as "soul-mating," comes from exchanging energy and fusing with one's partner.

How is it possible to turn the momentary orgasmic contractions into long-lasting states of ecstasy? It all begins with your arousal or sexual energy, which you have learned about in the last two chapters. As we discussed there, the expansion of our sexual energy (what we naively call "getting horny") is the secret to our sex life and our life itself. It is through sexual energy that we are conceived, and it is sexual energy that is the basis of our health, creativity, and joy, both in and out of bed.

Learning to cultivate your sexual energy will give you a sexual freedom that few people have: it will allow you to be sexual whenever you want and to circulate this powerful sexual energy to revitalize the rest of your life when you do not. Michael Winn, one of the Senior Universal Tao instructors, explains that sexual energy is available to us twenty-four hours a day, but most of us starve ourselves and believe that we can satisfy our needs for this healing energy with just a few minutes of intercourse. One of the most liberating realizations for people who practice Healing Love is that they have access to their sexual energy anytime and anywhere.

First, we must begin to understand what this sexual energy is (beyond some uncontrollable horniness or long-lost desire that comes and goes as it pleases). Then we can learn how it relates to the rest of our bodily energy and to our life as a whole.

One of the most liberating realizations for people who practice Healing Love is that they have access to their sexual energy anytime and anywhere.

Your Energy

As we mentioned in the Introduction, Healing Love, or Sexual Kung Fu, developed as part of Chinese medicine, which is one of the world's oldest healing systems and responsible for effective therapies such as acupuncture,

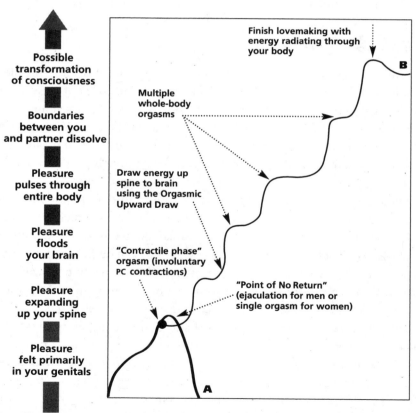

Possible transformation of consciousness

Boundaries between you and partner dissolve

Pleasure pulses through entire body

Pleasure floods your brain

Pleasure expanding up your spine

Pleasure felt primarily in your genitals

Finish lovemaking with energy radiating through your body

B

Multiple whole-body orgasms

Draw energy up spine to brain using the Orgasmic Upward Draw

"Contractile phase" orgasm (involuntary PC contractions)

"Point of No Return" (ejaculation for men or single orgasm for women)

A

Your Orgasmic Potential—instead of the ordinary ejaculatory orgasm for men or singular orgasm for women, you and your partner can multiply and expand your orgasms throughout your body.

A. Ordinary "Big Bang" ejaculatory orgasm for men or single orgasm for women
B. Multiple whole-body orgasm with Orgasmic Upward Draw

acupressure, and chi kung. Chinese medicine has long known that in addition to the structures of the body, there is a bioelectric energy, called *chi* (pronounced *CHEE*), that constantly circulates through every cell of our body. As Western physiology and chemistry have become more advanced, they have demonstrated that indeed our whole body and the whole universe is made of energy and electrical charges. As Dr. Felice Dunas explains, "Taking a number of different forms, chi flows constantly through our bodies, creating brain waves, causing the heart to beat, stimulating the nervous system, driving cell metabolism . . ."[1]

The recognition of our bodily energy, or chi, is not unique to China. The West may in fact be one of the few cultures that does not have a traditional term for this bioelectric energy, although even in the West we commonly speak of feeling *energized* or being *low energy*. The best way to understand chi, however, is not to explain it but to feel it in your own body.

Cultivating Your Energy

While Western science does not yet know why this energy, or chi, circulates on the paths that it does, Chinese medicine long ago mapped out these paths and learned to use them for greater health. You only need to learn the basic path along which energy travels in your body. It is called the Microcosmic Orbit (see illustration opposite), and it rises up from your sexual organs and travels along your spine up to your head and down through your tongue and the front of your body to your navel and back to your sexual organs.

These channels are not arbitrary. They arise from our earliest development in utero. When we are first conceived, our body resembles a flat disk, which then folds over. This leaves two "seams" along the back and front of the body. The back seam is easy to see in the spine. The front seam is less obvious. It can be seen when closure is not complete, as in children who are born with a harelip, or on many women during pregnancy when they develop a dark line up the center of their belly called the *linea nigra*.

The Microcosmic Orbit is really two channels: one that goes up your back and one that comes down your front. It is your tongue that actually connects the two channels, closing the circuit. *So it is essential that you learn to touch the tip of your tongue to the front roof of your mouth* (see illustration on p. 70). There is a little indentation at the front of the roof of your mouth (your palate), and it is through here that the energy descends most easily from your brain and moves through your tongue and down your throat and chest to your abdomen.

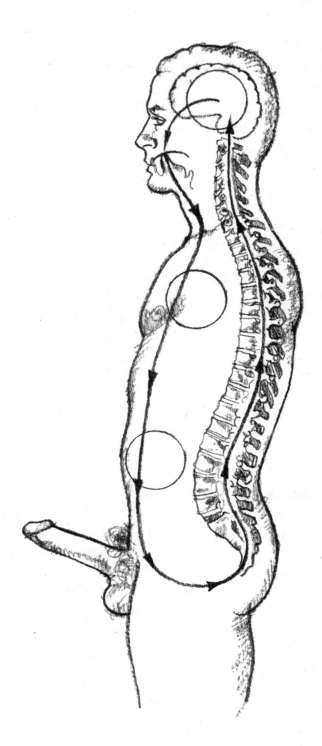

The Microcosmic Orbit—a natural circuit of energy in the body. There are three reservoirs of energy, at the brain, heart, and abdomen.

(If you have high blood pressure, you should keep your tongue in your lower jaw rather than touching your palate, and also make sure to bring the energy all the way down to the soles of your feet.)

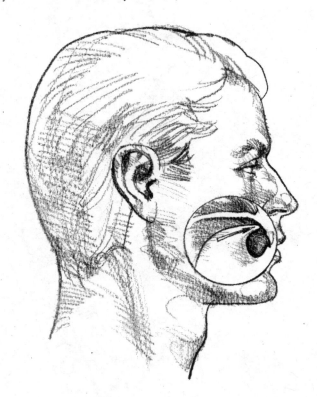

Touching your tongue to your palate

FEELING ENERGY MOVE IN YOUR BODY

Many people are surprised to learn that they have energy moving in their body all the time, but like the invisible bonds of atoms that hold our world together, it is always, if silently, present. Without it, we would not be alive. Usually we are not aware of this energy, which is subtle and constantly moving, but as we cultivate it, we can learn to move it with our mind and to experience its warm, tingling feeling throughout our body for greater pleasure and health.

What Does Energy Feel Like When It Is Moving in My Body? Warmth and tingling are two feelings that many people describe. Others feel prickling (like static electricity), pulsating, humming, bubbling, or buzzing. Most people feel it move slowly, especially at first, almost like molasses. While it sometimes can move quickly, like a rush of energy, it is very important not to try to force it. Don't be surprised if you feel the energy more at some places than at others.

How Can I Move Energy? There is an old Taoist saying, "The mind moves and the chi follows." Wherever you focus your attention, the chi tends to gather and increase. This fact has been demonstrated through biofeedback experiments that indicate increased activity in the nerves and muscles in the area where a person focuses attention. You can test this through an experiment. Concentrate on warming your hands, and notice how the blood and chi flow to your hands. It is this awareness of the power of the mind to affect our body that the Western technique of biofeedback uses to help people control their body's seemingly unconscious processes.

Remember: you are not pushing or pulling the chi; you are simply shifting your focus to another place. This is very important because you do not want to force the energy, which can cause you to hurt yourself. Energy is very powerful, and you need to move it slowly and gently. In fact, it is much easier to move energy if your body is soft and relaxed than if it is rigid and tense.

You are not pushing or pulling the chi; you are simply shifting your focus to another place.

Sexual Energy

Sexual energy, or *ching-chi* (pronounced CHING-CHEE), is a very powerful form of bioelectric energy. When you get aroused, or horny, it is this spreading of sexual energy that you are feeling in your body. As we have discussed above, Healing Love is based on developing the ability to cultivate this sexual energy for your pleasure, health, and spiritual growth. In the Orgasmic Upward Draw exercise, we will show you how to draw the sexual energy up out of your genitals and circulate it through the rest of your body. According to the Taoists, since we are conceived through orgasm and orgasmic energy permeates every cell of our body, we need to feel this rejuvenating, orgasmic energy regularly—ideally every day—to stay healthy.

When you are able to circulate this energy, you will find that you have a great deal more energy. Indeed, when you are able to draw up your sexual energy to your brain, you will find that it is more effective than caffeine for giving you a shot of energy when you are feeling tired. Unlike with caffeine, however, there are no side effects.

According to the Taoists, since we are conceived through orgasm and orgasmic energy permeates every cell of our body, we need to feel this rejuvenating, orgasmic energy regularly— ideally every day—to stay healthy.

In the exhausting rush of our modern life, juggling work and family, we often have very little energy left for lovemaking. Yet it is lovemaking, when done with the healing circulation of energy, that can rejuvenate us more than any artificial stimulant.

Generating, Transforming, and Storing Sexual Energy

Before you learn to circulate your sexual energy up to your brain, you will need to learn how to bring the energy already in your brain down to your abdomen. As we discussed, our genitals are capable of generating an enormous amount of energy (you certainly know this!), but this part of our body is not good at using or storing this energy. Our brain, on the other hand, is superb at transforming and projecting this energy out into the world through our thinking and creativity. The brain, however, is not very good at generating or storing energy. For this reason, it is never good to leave energy in the brain for very long. The energy should always be brought down to the abdomen, for it is the organs in our abdomen that are ideal for storing energy. The organs store and release energy to the body when it is needed, almost like timed-release capsules. As we will discuss in chapter 5, for the Taoists, bringing orgasmic energy to our organs is a vital part of maintaining our health.

Finding the Way

Energy in the Body

- GENITALS: Generate energy

- BRAIN: Transforms and projects energy

- ORGANS: Store energy

WHAT GOES UP MUST COME DOWN

One of the major differences between the Taoist sexual practices and the Tantric sexual practices of India is how the energy is channeled through the body. In Tantra, sexual energy is channeled from the root chakra (or energy point at the genitals) up to the brain. This can be a profound and even mind-alerting experience, but it can also lead to painful or dangerous amounts of energy in the brain. According to the Taoists, who modeled their practices on the natural world, "what goes up must come down." For this reason, the Taoists know it is essential to bring energy that one circulates to one's brain back down to the navel, where it can be safely stored and where the body can absorb it more easily.

WHAT DOES YOUR GUT TELL YOU?

Modern people spend most of their energy in their brain. Our information civilization requires constant mental energy, and many of us can get stuck in our head. Bringing the energy down from our head to our abdomen allows us to store the energy safely and to have more energy available to fuel our sex life and our desire for life.

There is another reason why it is important to bring energy down, and the Taoists knew this also. In our abdomen resides another center of intelligence in the body, which might be called our "second brain" or "feeling brain."

Today, we tend to think that all of our thoughts and feelings originate in our head. The Taoists, however, saw feelings as energies that arise from different organs and not just from the brain. This is also part of common knowledge in the West. We have long associated the emotion of love with the heart. We now know that in addition to our brain there are other nerve centers at our heart, our solar plexus, and our abdomen.

There is startling new evidence that the extent and complexity of the neural web in the abdomen approach those of the brain. Researchers are now calling this the "abdominal brain." In colloquial speech we recognize this, as we often say, "My gut tells me . . ." or "My gut feelings are . . ." This gut-level knowledge is often considered more intuitive and more accurate. The Taoists were particularly interested in the potential of the abdominal brain because it uses less energy than the brain in our head to do the same "thinking."

You will now learn how to bring the energy down to your abdomen through the Inner Smile. This will allow your body to use it when necessary. As you bring the energy down to your abdomen, direct it to your navel. Your navel is more than just the vestigial scar of your umbilical cord. According to the Taoists, the navel is where all nourishment flows into our body in utero, and it remains the *energetic center* of our body.

Finally, the Inner Smile is the first step of the Orgasmic Upward Draw. As it is necessary to empty a glass before it can be filled, drawing energy down from your brain with the Inner Smile will allow your brain to fill up again with fresh rejuvenating energy from your genitals.

> It is essential to bring energy that one circulates to one's brain back down to the navel, where it can be safely stored and where the body can absorb it more easily.

Drawing energy down from your brain with the Inner Smile will allow your brain to fill up again with fresh rejuvenating energy from your genitals.

THE INNER SMILE

The Inner Smile is an extremely simple but powerful exercise. It was just like the Taoists, who tried to align themselves with nature, to notice the profound impact of something as simple and ordinary as a smile. We tend to think that when we are happy we smile. But there is compelling research that suggests the opposite is also true. When we smile, we feel happier as well, even if we did not begin by feeling good. All of us have experienced the power of a smile: we can recall a time when we were sad or sick and someone, possibly even a stranger, gave us a big smile, and immediately we felt better. The Taoists have long known the profound energetic and healing power of smiling.

The Taoists would say that when you smile, your organs release powerful secretions that nourish the whole body. On the other hand, when you are angry, fearful, or under stress, your organs produce toxic secretions that block the energy channels, settling in the organs and causing loss of appetite, indigestion, increased blood pressure, faster heartbeat, insomnia, and negative emotions. While the presence of such secretions has not been demonstrated clinically, the connection between stress and illness is well established in the medical literature. Smiling and cultivating joy and happiness are important for your overall well-being and for a healthy love life.

Finding the Way

Smiling Eyes

The Taoists noticed a very interesting point about smiling. Real smiling comes not just from the mouth but also from the eyes. "Smiling eyes" is an expression in English, and it conveys the essence of this insight. When we truly smile, we do so with both our lips and our eyes. When you smile, try to soften the corners of both your mouth and your eyes, smiling from both.

The Inner Smile will also cultivate your love and compassion, which is an essential part of working with your sexual energy. As we will discuss in chapter 6, for healing lovemaking it is essential to keep lust connected to love, or in other words to keep the sexual energy in our genitals connected with the compassionate energy of our heart. Since sexual energy simply magnifies whatever emotions you are feeling, it is essential that you *not* practice (or

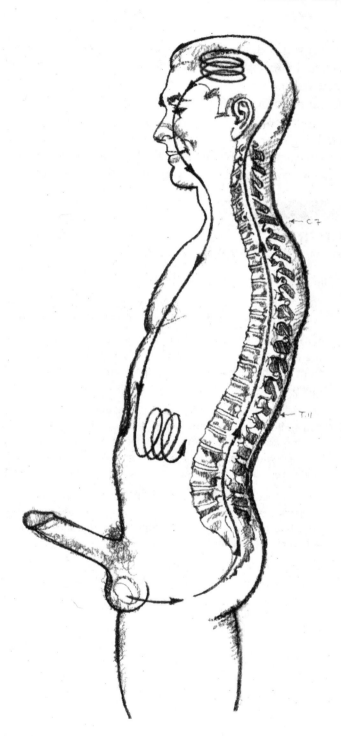

*Inner Smile—
bringing energy down
to your abdomen
helps you empty
energy from your
head, so that it can be
replenished with
sexual energy rising
along the spine.*

make love) when you are feeling anger or other strong negative emotions. Whenever you have sex, your attitude should be one of joy and love both for yourself and for your partner. In addition, try to smile and be playful as you circulate your energy.

Do not be surprised if it takes you a little while to feel the energy come down to your abdomen. Men especially often find it easier to draw energy up than to bring it down. You may simply need to circulate more sexual energy before you can feel it descend down the front of your body. The exercise after this will give you plenty of energy to work with—or play with. Enjoy.

Exercise 13

INNER SMILE
DRAWING YOUR ENERGY DOWN

1.   RELAX: Relax and breathe deeply.

2.   TOUCH NAVEL: Touch your navel with your fingertips, gently pulling it open. (This will activate your navel and help you bring energy down.)

3.   TOUCH TONGUE TO ROOF OF MOUTH: Touch the tip of your tongue to the front roof of your mouth (see illustration on p. 70) to connect the front and back channels of your body and to allow the energy to flow down from your head to your abdomen.

4.   SMILE DOWN TO YOUR NAVEL: Smile as you focus on your navel. When you smile, soften the corners of your lips and your eyes. Feel the sun shining down on you, and as you smile feel warm energy descending through your head and torso down to your navel. Let the energy gather there. You can spiral the energy around your navel to help it absorb.

5.   TOUCH FINGERTIPS TO YOUR HEART: Then touch your heart with your fingertips and smile as you focus on your heart and on making it soft. As your heart softens, you can imagine it opening like a red flower blossoming with love and compassion.

6.   BRING ENERGY TO ABDOMEN: Keep smiling and then bring this loving and compassionate energy back down to the abdomen.

Orgasmic Upward Draw

After bringing the energy down with the Inner Smile, you will then bring the energy up with the Orgasmic Upward Draw. Bringing the sexual energy in your genitals up your spine will allow you to experience a refreshing, revitalizing wave of energy up your spine, stimulating all the nerves of the body along the way. During lovemaking, this ability to draw sexual energy up will allow you to expand your genital orgasms into whole-body orgasms. Eventually, as you cultivate your ability to circulate energy, you can feel this orgasmic wave of pleasure at any time without even having to be sexual. Now *that's* better than a double latte.

Learning to circulate this energy down and then up may take some time, so do not be discouraged. On the other hand, you may find that you are able to move the energy almost immediately. Much will depend on your bodily awareness and your concentration. Do not be concerned if you do not feel much during the first few days or weeks of practice. If this is your first time practicing meditation, yoga, or martial arts, it will take you longer to learn the practice. Soon, however, you will be surprised how easily the energy moves. Since the energy flows along natural circuits in your body, the energy will guide your mind even as your mind is trying to guide the energy.

Your genitals are a powerful source of energy. You are learning to tap into their energy and circulate it along the circuits of your body to revitalize you. The ancient Taoist metaphor compared our body's energy to water. Your genitals and spine are like a water wheel that draws the energy up your spine and then pours it into your head to replenish your brain. From there it flows down like a waterfall into your abdomen, where it can be stored in a life-giving reservoir of energy. The Taoists knew that there is nothing more powerful in nature than water and nothing more powerful in our body than our sexual energy. So it is essential that you learn to use it safely.

Since the energy flows along natural circuits in your body, the energy will guide your mind even as your mind is trying to guide the energy.

Orgasmic Upward Draw—man drawing sexual energy from his genitals up to the crown of his head

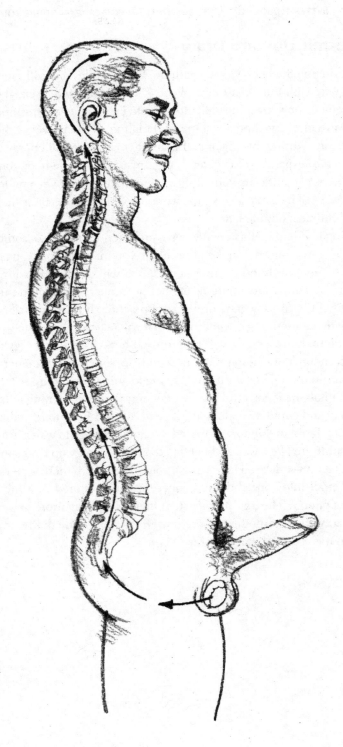

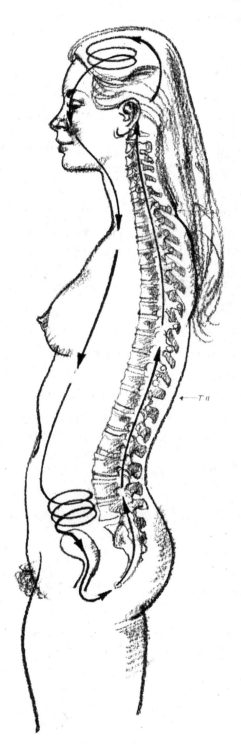

T II

Inner Smile and Orgasmic Upward Draw—woman bringing energy down with Inner Smile and then drawing energy up to the crown of her head with Orgasmic Upward Draw

Finding the Way

Cautions

The Orgasmic Upward Draw is a very powerful practice, and you need to make sure you follow a few safety tips.

NEVER LEAVE SEXUAL ENERGY IN YOUR HEAD FOR LONG PERIODS OF TIME

Remember to bring the energy down from your brain to your abdomen, where it can be safely stored. In the past, many teachers of Eastern sexuality taught students how to draw energy up to the brain without teaching them how to bring it back down again. This resulted in what has been called the "Kundalini Syndrome." The Taoists knew the importance of completing the energetic circle. Anytime you feel you have too much energy in your head, you should do the Inner Smile to bring the energy down to your abdomen. If you feel like you still have too much energy in your body, you can always do Exercise 16: Bringing Energy Down, on page 86, or Exercise 17: Venting, on page 88. Looking down with your eyes and focusing on your feet will also help bring the energy down.

HIGH BLOOD PRESSURE WARNING

If you have high blood pressure, you should keep your tongue in your lower jaw rather than touching your palate, and also make sure to bring the energy all the way down to the soles of your feet.

MAKE SURE YOU ARE HEALTHY

Remember, the sexual energy is powerful. If you have a serious medical condition, you should speak with a Universal Tao instructor (see Resources) before you begin this practice. If you have an active herpes sore, do not do this practice until you have healed. If you have herpes but it is in remission (that is, if you have no visible sore), you can do this practice.

TAKE IT EASY

Your attitude toward the practice is essential. You need to make sure that you are relaxed and playful with the energy. Don't try to force it up your spine or around your body, or you can hurt yourself.

PREPARE YOURSELF

Practice on an empty but not hungry stomach whenever possible. Always wait at least an hour after eating. The body needs energy to digest the food you have eaten, which means there will be less energy for you to circulate. Also, wear loose clothes. Although there should be a gentle flow of clean air in the room, avoid drafts or wind. And remember to always breathe through your nose.

POSITION

In the beginning, do not lie on your back during these exercises, since the rising sexual energy may stick in your chest and cause pain. At first, sit, stand, or lie on your side (preferably your right side). Once you master these exercises, you can do them in any position. Also, never place any objects (such as a pillow) under you while lying on your side, since this will bend the channel of energy and could cause pain.

ORGASMIC UPWARD DRAW
DRAWING YOUR ENERGY UP

1. **BRING ENERGY TO GENITALS:** Now that you have learned to bring energy down with the Inner Smile, you are ready to draw it up. From your abdomen move your hands down to cover your pelvis. Smile and bring the energy down to your sexual organs. Be aware of the sun above you, and feel the energy from the sun and from your smiling eyes warming up your sexual organs. You can also touch your genitals to increase the sexual energy, or if you are in a public place you can simply think of a sexual thought.

2. **CONTRACT YOUR PC MUSCLE, PERINEUM, AND ANUS:** Once you feel a slight tingling or stirring of your sexual energy, *very gently contract your PC muscle, perineum, and anus.* Doing this will draw the energy from the sexual organs into the sacrum (or tailbone) and lower spine.

3. **LET ENERGY RISE TO YOUR HEAD:** Let the energy rise up the spine to the brain. Gently tucking your chin in will help the energy move from your spine into your head.

4. **SPIRAL THE ENERGY IN YOUR HEAD:** Spiral the energy in your head using your mind and eyes. Circle nine times in one direction and nine times in the other direction. This will help your brain to absorb this creative sexual energy.

5. **STORE ENERGY IN YOUR ABDOMEN:** Touch your navel again, touch your tongue to the roof of your mouth, and smile back down to the navel with your mouth and eyes. The energy will return from your brain to the abdomen, where it can be stored in the organs.

While each step in the Orgasmic Upward Draw will help you draw the energy up, the most important part of the practice is *contracting your PC and anus because it is this squeezing action that literally pumps the energy up the spine.* Soon you will be able to draw the energy up to your head using simply your mind and possibly a squeeze of your anus. At first, however, you may need to draw the energy up your spine gradually and slowly.

You also may find that you feel the energy at certain points along your spine more than at others. This is natural, as some parts of your spine may be more flexible than others. If your back or pelvis is tight it will be difficult for you to draw sexual energy up through your spine.

Finding the Way

Loosening Up

You can loosen up your spine easily by sitting at the edge of a chair and rocking your pelvis from side to side. Rock from your hips, like a belly dancer. Smile and rock your lower spine, middle spine, and upper spine.

Once you have learned to do the Inner Smile and the Orgasmic Upward Draw, you will be able to circulate the energy easily in any situation, while you are walking around, standing in line at the grocery store, driving your car, or lying in bed. While to the world it may look like you are participating in the chores of everyday life, you are actually cultivating your sexual energy and feeling blissful waves of orgasmic energy.

I Don't Feel My Sexual Energy We have suggested that you do the Orgasmic Upward Draw when your sexual energy is not too aroused. The hotter it is, the more difficult it is to control. For men, this means that they are more likely to ejaculate, losing the energy they are trying to draw up. However, if you do not feel enough sexual energy, arouse yourself 50 to 70 percent of the way to orgasm. Women, and men who have learned to separate orgasm from ejaculation, can arouse themselves all the way to orgasm and still draw the energy up to their brain. When you are about to orgasm or are orgasming, stop and do the Orgasmic Upward Draw three to nine times, or until the orgasmic feeling moves upward.

I Can't Raise the Energy up My Spine If you are having problems drawing the energy up your spine, you can help the energy rise by using your spine's natural pumps. Your cerebrospinal fluid bathes the brain and spine. Pumps at your sacrum (the back of your pelvis) and the base of the skull help this fluid circulate and can also help you draw energy up your spine. These pumps, which are used by osteopathic physicians today, were well known to the ancient Taoists. You can do the following exercises standing or sitting.

Exercise 15

PUMPING THE ENERGY UP

1. ROCK YOUR PELVIS: Activate your sacral pump by squeezing your anus up toward your tailbone and rocking your pelvis back and forth as if you are riding a horse.

2. DRAW IN YOUR CHIN: Activate your cranial pump (at the base of your skull) by drawing your chin in and up and then back out in a soft gentle circle. Keep the jaw and neck muscles relaxed.

3. DRAW THE ENERGY UP YOUR SPINE: After activating the sacral and cranial pumps, rest and begin drawing the energy up your spine into your brain. Looking up with your eyes toward the top of your head will also help direct the energy up to the crown of your head. Repeatedly activate these pumps until you feel the energy move up.

My Back Hurts It is sometimes a little difficult to draw the energy into the base of the spine, and some people experience a little pain, tingling, or pins and needles when this energy first enters their spine. If this happens to you, do not be alarmed. You can help pass the energy through by gently massaging the area with your fingers.

My Eyes Hurt When you roll your eyes around to circulate the energy, you may find your eye muscles ache or your head aches. This is a typical sign of sore muscles (we rarely use our eye muscles deliberately) and is nothing to worry about. If this problem persists, roll your eyes less and use more mental focus to circulate the energy.

My Head Hurts If your head hurts, you feel wired, or you are having difficulty sleeping, you may be leaving too much stagnant energy in your head. The energy can overheat if it stays in one place—a problem that can be easily solved by keeping the energy moving. Make sure to circulate the energy in your head nine, eighteen, or thirty-six times in one direction and then the other. Once you have circled the energy in your head, let it flow down the front of your body.

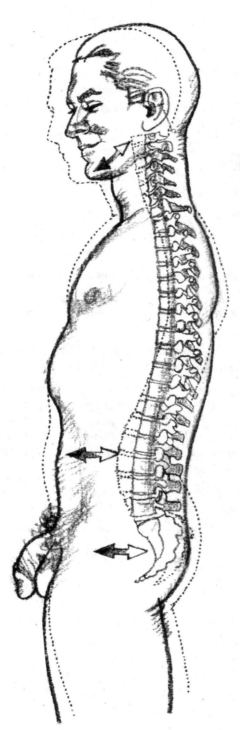

Sacral and Cranial Pumps—you can help your energy rise by rocking your pelvis and drawing your chin in.

What If I Can't Bring the Energy Down?   Sometimes people who spend a lot of time "in their head" find they have a difficult time bringing the energy down. As a result, they may find they have difficulty sleeping or find that they are a little wired by this additional energy, as if they had too much caffeine. Remember the brain is excellent for transforming and using energy, but it is not very good for storing energy. It is best to bring the excess energy down to your abdomen. The following exercise will help.

Exercise 16

BRINGING ENERGY DOWN

1.   **HANDS ON ABDOMEN:** Place your hands on your abdomen.

2.   **TONGUE TO FRONT OF PALATE:** Touch your tongue to the front of your palate, as shown on p. 70.

3.   **SMILE:** Smile, gently curving your lips up and smiling with the corners of your eyes.

4.   **RELAX:** Relax your body, and release any tension or blockages you may feel.

5.   **FOCUS ON YOUR ABDOMEN:** Bring your attention down to your navel (remember the energy will follow your focus).

6.   **BRING THE ENERGY DOWN:** Imagine the energy descending down the front of your body like a waterfall and pooling in your abdomen. Cup your left hand within your right just below your belly button, as if you were catching the waterfall of energy. Alternatively, imagine the energy is like molasses or honey being drawn down and wound around a spiral at your belly button.

7.   **SWALLOW YOUR SALIVA:** Swallowing your saliva can also help you draw the energy down.

If you are still having problems bringing the energy down, you can use Exercise 17: Venting, on p. 88.

I Am Feeling Angry and Irritable   In addition to amplifying anger that you may already have, the new energy can also cause you to overheat and develop negative emotions, such as anger or impatience, if you are not circulating the energy enough. In this case try to focus on recycling the anger and negative emotions into loving-kindness (see Exercise 24: Recycling Our Negative Emotions, on p. 163). It is also very important to remember to smile and to bring the energy down. If you find you are prone to feel certain negative emotions, you can cultivate these emotions and recycle this energy by following the Six Healing Sounds in Mantak Chia's *Taoist Secrets for Transforming Stress into Vitality.*

OTHER SIDE EFFECTS

Very rarely a person may experience excess energy stuck in the upper body. Symptoms of this vary from person to person but may include insomnia, a ringing in the ears, heart palpitations, or tension headaches that persist for several days. If you have any of these symptoms, immediately stop the practice and do the Venting exercise. If they persist, contact a Universal Tao instructor (see the Resources) or acupuncturist. Most Western doctors will not be able to correctly diagnose or treat the problem since they are not trained to understand the movement of energy in the body and its physical effects. It is worth mentioning that the problems are not caused by circulating your sexual energy but by preexisting emotional and physical tensions trapped in the upper body. The sexual energy simply amplifies these existing problems, which is why it is essential for you to address these underlying issues before advancing further with your sexual practice.

ABSORBING THE ENERGY

After each time that you practice the Orgasmic Upward Draw, you may wish to massage your genital area gently to help absorb any sexual energy that did not get drawn up. This will reduce any feelings of congestion or fullness in this part of your body. Men in particular often experience pressure in their testicles when they begin or if they have not circulated all of their sexual energy. Gently rubbing their testicles between their thumb and fingers as well as massaging their perineum and tailbone will help relieve these feelings of fullness. If you feel the energy is getting stuck anywhere in your body, you can help it keep moving and get absorbed by stroking or massaging the area.

After a month or more of practice, you may find that you feel some pressure in your head, which is a result of the increased energy in your body. This is a sign of progress, that your body has more energy than before. Most people experience this as pleasurable tingling. However, if this additional energy grows uncomfortable, make sure that you are bringing it down to your abdomen. Physical exercise, massaging your feet, and a heavy grain diet can all help to ground the energy. Having an orgasm without circulating the energy and, for men, ejaculating will also help reduce this energy.

With this energy, however, you will find that you need less sleep and have more energy for your life, for your relationship, and for cultivating your physical, emotional, intellectual, and spiritual life, which was the true goal of the Tao and the true gift of Healing Love.

Exercise 17

VENTING

1. Sit in a chair or lie down on your back. If lying down, elevate your knees with a pillow if you feel any pain in the small of your back or lumbar area.

2. Place your hands in front of your mouth so that the tips of your fingers touch and so that your palms are facing toward your feet.

3. Close your eyes and take a deep breath. Feel your stomach and chest expand gently.

4. Smile and exhale quietly, making the sound *heeeeee.* As you are exhaling, push your hands toward your feet. Picture your body as a hollow tube of blue light that you are emptying with your hands from your head down past your chest and your abdomen, through your legs and out the soles of your feet.

5. Repeat the sound and movement three, six, or nine times. If you are still having a problem venting your energy, contact a Universal Tao instructor (see the Resources) or an acupuncturist.

Understanding the Power of Your Sexual Energy

It is vital that you understand how powerful your sexual energy is and how important it is to cultivate and refine it. Because it is so important we will mention several times throughout the book that expanding your sexual energy will simply expand whatever energy and emotions you have in your body—positive or negative. If you feel love, expanding your sexual energy will expand this love. However, if you feel anger or even hate, expanding your sexual energy will expand these emotions as well.

This is no doubt a major reason why the techniques for expanding our sexual energy were closely guarded secrets and why so many religions have been

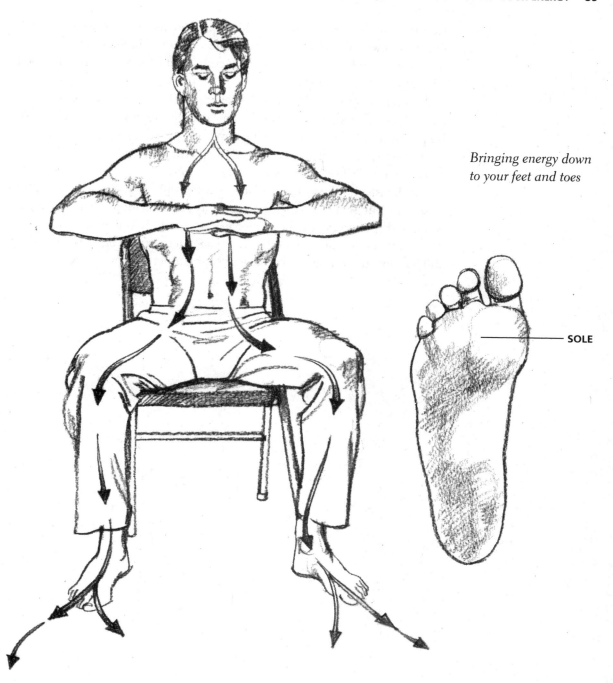

*Bringing energy down
to your feet and toes*

SOLE

fearful about the power of our sexuality. The Tao does not believe in controlling this powerful energy through shame or denial. Rather, it believes we must understand its power and learn to cultivate it for our good and the good of others.

As you learn to expand your sexual energy, make sure that you read chapters 5, 6, and 7, which will show you how to cultivate this energy and how to keep your sex life filled with healing, love, and compassion. In particular, do not forget to practice Exercise 24: Recycling Our Negative Emotions, p. 163, and Exercise 27: The Compassion Cycle, p. 174.

For Taoists, however, the physical is always primary. So, first, we must begin with our bodies and their extraordinary potential for pleasure. Now that you have begun to explore how you can each multiply and expand your own individual orgasms, we will discuss how you can share this orgasmic pleasure and harmonize your desire with that of your partner.

PART TWO

Duo:

Sharing Passion,

Healing, and Intimacy

with Your Partner

CHAPTER 4

Pleasuring Each Other

In this chapter you will discover:

- How to Harmonize Male and Female Desire and Satisfy Each Other Fully

- The Art of Fingering and the Art of Stroking

- The G Spot and Other Vaginal Spots

- The Art of Cunnilingus and the Art of Fellatio

- The Art of Taoist Thrusting

In this chapter you will learn how to pleasure each other and how to harmonize your desire for more profound and satisfying lovemaking. The Taoists understood the fundamental differences that often exist between male and female sexuality. They also recognized that harmony in the bedroom and happiness in relationships were dependent on each partner knowing the needs of the other. The Taoist doctors were early sexologists, and they observed every aspect of male and female sexuality to discover their secrets and their satisfactions.

Before we discuss some of the differences that often exist between male and female sexuality, we want to emphasize that every person's desire is unique. The generalities that follow about desire will need to be qualified by your and your partner's actual experiences. Remember, you do not need to become the best lover in the world, just the best lover of your own partner. Let your partner's desire and pleasure guide you.

You do not need to become the best lover in the world, just the best lover of your own partner.

Fire and Water

The Taoists compared male sexuality to fire and female sexuality to water. While male sexuality is easily ignited (men get aroused easily), it is also easily extinguished (men ejaculate quickly). Female sexuality, although slower to bring to a boil (women take longer to get aroused), is the stronger and more long lasting of the two (women don't end with ejaculation and are slower to cool down).

The Taoists compared male sexuality to fire and female sexuality to water.

The Taoists knew that these differences in male and female sexuality are the cause of much discontent in the bedroom, and they sought to harmonize male and female sexuality. By teaching men how to bring women's desire to a rapid boil before and during intercourse, they knew that there was a much greater likelihood that men and women would crescendo together. By teaching men to delay ejaculation and have multiple orgasms like women, they knew that men and women could ride many peaks of pleasure together for the most satisfying and healing lovemaking.

Men Are from Yang, Women Are from Yin

Before you can understand how to harmonize male and female sexuality, you need to understand why men and women often have such different sexual needs. According to the Tao, men are primarily *yang*, which means that they have mostly yang, or masculine energy. This energy is one of the two primordial forces of the universe and has many associated qualities, one of them being quickness to action, or, in this case, arousal. Women are primarily *yin*, which means that they have mostly yin, or feminine energy. This energy is the other primordial force of the universe and has many associated qualities, one of them being slowness to action, or, in this case, arousal.

In the words of Taoist master Wu Hsien from two thousand years ago:

> Male belongs to Yang.
> Yang's uniqueness is that he gets aroused quickly.
> But he quickly retreats.
> Female belongs to Yin.
> Yin's uniqueness is that she is slower to be aroused,
> But she is also slow to retreat.

Yin and yang, for Taoists, are the two complementary and cyclical forces in the universe that create everything. Positive and negative in charge, they are both essential and mutually interdependent. Each person has both masculine and feminine energy, and yin and yang can actually change into each other. This may explain the complexity and variability of our individual desire.

It is important to remember that there are some women who are more yang than yin, whom we will call "yangful women," and there are some men who have more yin than yang, whom we will call "yinful men." In addition, our work, our diet, and our life as a whole affect our energetic balance. In this discussion, we necessarily need to make generalizations, but you should adapt them to your and your partner's own sexuality.

If you are a yangful woman, you may find your experience is more equivalent to that of most men. If you are a yinful man, you may find your experience is more equivalent to that of most women. While for convenience we divide into two broad categories, our sexuality and sexual energy really lie on a spectrum.

While individually unique, men tend to have far more yang energy and women tend to have far more yin. As gender roles have changed over the past fifty years, this has changed somewhat, but the energetic differences in yin and yang remain, just as there remain fundamental hormonal differences between men and women. Indeed, hormonal research over the past ten years seems to echo this several-thousand-year-old Taoist understanding.[1]

Each person has both masculine and feminine energy, and yin and yang can actually change into each other.

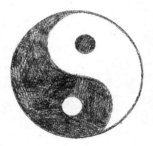

According to the Tao, yin and yang are the two complementary forces in the universe that represent feminine and masculine energies.

Arousal: Boiling Water and Igniting a Flame

Yin moves downward—like water—trickling through a woman's body from her head to her heart and finally to her genitals.

Understanding how yin and yang work in our body can also explain the different ways that men and women get aroused. As acupuncturist Felice Dunas, Ph.D., points out in her excellent book, *Passion Play*, yin moves downward—like water—trickling through a woman's body from her head to her heart and finally to her genitals. This, she explains, is why most women need to have their head and heart opened before they can open up sexually. This slow movement of energy down her body is also why a woman tends to need more foreplay and time spent caressing and coaxing her energy away from distracting thoughts and emotions and into her genitals.

Yang moves up—like fire—from a man's genitals to his heart and head.

Yang, on the other hand, moves up—like fire—from a man's genitals to his heart and head. This is why men get aroused much more quickly than women and tend to need much less foreplay. As a result, most men can be aroused by direct genital approach. For them, this *is* foreplay.

We tend to say that men are much more "genitally focused," which is based on the fact that their sexual energy begins in their genitals. As it rises and spreads throughout their body through lovemaking, they are much more able to connect with their heart and receive their partner's love. When a man ejaculates quickly, however, all of his sexual energy spills out without rising up through his body. The sexual energy never reaches his heart, and the sex never really becomes "lovemaking" for him. As a man learns to have a whole-body orgasm and to circulate his energy, it rises up to his heart and brain, allowing him to expand his love for his partner. This is the real secret of making *love* for men.

This difference in arousal has caused countless generations of misunderstanding and sexual disharmony in the bedroom. We can regret it and resent it, but understanding it is the surest way to mutual satisfaction.

In the following section, we will describe several secrets for harmonizing desire between men and women. Keep in mind that if your sexual lives are already in harmony, you may not need all the following suggestions. Certainly, you will not need to follow every step each time.

Harmonizing Your Desires

The first part of harmonizing your desires is being aware of the differences between you, whatever they may be. In general, men will need to control their flame to stay with their partner while heating up their partner's waters through skillful sexual foreplay. Women can help most by sparking their own desire. The Taoists recommended couples focus first on arousing the woman and bringing her desire to a rapid boil. However, arousal (for both partners) begins long before you reach the bedroom.

PREHEAT YOUR PARTNER

Just like an oven, which gets hotter when preheated, so our desire should also be turned on in advance. Igniting the thought of lovemaking before falling into bed will ensure that you fall into each other's arms instead of falling asleep. Calling each other during the day and sharing your desire for each other that night works wonders for getting the sensual imagination working. Tantalizing each other during the evening with loving words and caresses can get the flame of passion burning bright by the time you go to bed.

While this is valuable for both partners, it is essential for many women. There is an old cliché that women want romance and men want sex. Both men and women want sex; women often just need more romance to awaken their sexual energy and bring it down into their genitals. While men also need to have their passion ignited, their firelike sexual energy is a pilot light that generally responds more quickly. According to the Tao, there is no judgment in these differences. The Tao seeks to understand life, not to judge it.

PREPARING THE SACRED CHAMBER

Having sex in various rooms of the house or in unusual places is fun and can add spontaneity and variety to your sex life. The Taoists were great fans of making love outside, close to the natural world that they revered and tried to emulate. Most sex, however, happens in the bedroom, so it is important to make sure that you have a sex-friendly bedroom.

Our body is deeply affected by the sights, sounds, and smells that surround it. When we create a space that looks and feels safe and sensual, our body is unconsciously prepared for lovemaking. There is an old joke that women need a reason; men just need a place. The place, the suggestion is, could be anywhere. But both women's and men's bodies are influenced by the place that they are in and respond to familiar romantic rituals.

How romantic is your bedroom? Does it prepare you and your partner for lovemaking? How, you may ask, does a room prepare you for lovemaking? Just like a fine restaurant prepares you for a romantic meal. There is a beautiful

Tantalizing each other during the evening with loving words and caresses can start the flame of passion burning bright by the time you go to bed.

How romantic is your bedroom? Does it prepare you and your partner for lovemaking?

decor and soft lighting. Everyone has his or her own aesthetic of what feels nurturing and romantic, but make sure that your room nurtures and relaxes your bodies.

Keep distractions like books, papers, and television to a minimum. Sleep experts recommend that people who have difficulty sleeping avoid reading or watching television in bed. The rationale is the same. If we are accustomed to reading or watching television in a room, our body prepares for these activities rather than for sleep or, in our case, sex. If your television is the most prominent object in your bedroom, you will probably be watching it a lot more than you will be doing it. In short, try to keep your television out of your bedroom.

Lighting is also essential. While many people choose to make love in the dark, it is easiest to experience Healing Love when there is some, preferably soft, light. During Healing Love, couples focus their love and attention on each other's eyes and body. It is harder to be fully present with your partner when you are groping for each other in the dark.

Every body, whatever its shape and size, can be a source of energetic and ecstatic lovemaking.

Lighting a candle is an easy and regular ritual that can prepare your body for lovemaking. Candlelight allows us to gaze into each other's eyes and to rejoice in the lines and curves of our magnificent forms. Candlelight is also generous light, softening our shapes and hiding the imperfections that exist in all bodies. The focus of Healing Love is the subtle exchange of energy; it transcends the obsessions of body image that consume most modern people. Every body, whatever its shape and size, can be a source of energetic and ecstatic lovemaking.

Learning the Circuits of the Body

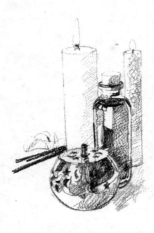

Our bodies are deeply affected by the sights, sounds, and smells that surround them.

Touching each other out of bed and in bed is vitally important to harmonizing desire and pleasuring each other. While touch is instinctual, most people do not know how or why touch is so important, and most people do not touch each other nearly enough.

When we touch each other, a hormone called oxytocin is released into our bloodstream, which increases our affection for each other, decreases our stress, and increases our production of sex hormones. For women it increases their sexual responsiveness, and for men it increases the sensitivity of their penis and improves their erection.[2]

Without regular affectionate touch women tend to become depressed and uninterested in sexual touch, while men tend to become more aggressive and become uninterested in touch that is not sexual—a recipe for marital disharmony if ever there was one. Holding hands and holding each other are not only emotionally satisfying; they also are physiologically essential.

In addition, our hormones create positive feedback loops, which means that the more you have it the more you want it. This is why the more touch we have the more we welcome touch, and the more sex we have the more open to sex we become.

Without regular touch women tend to become depressed and uninterested in sexual touch, while men tend to become more aggressive and become uninterested in touch that is not sexual—a recipe for marital disharmony if ever there was one.

Touch releases a hormone that increases our affection, our sexual responsiveness, and our sexual sensitivity.

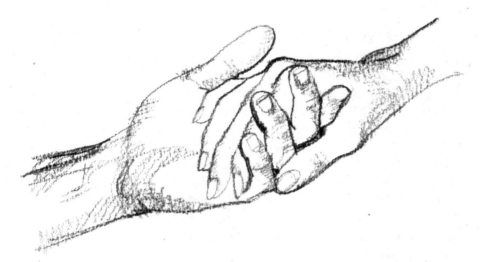

Unfortunately, the negative feedback loop is equally powerful, which is why couples enter into vicious cycles of separation in which they don't touch and don't make love. For this reason, it is important to continue touching each other even when you do not wish to be sexual.

It is also worth erring in the direction of having sex, assuming that there is no major reason not to (tiredness doesn't count). Because we are creatures of habit, if we do something today, we are more likely to do something tomorrow. In the case of sex, habit as well as hormones can encourage us. Keep the feedback loop moving in the right direction.

YOUR TOUCH IS ELECTRIC

For Taoists, touch is not simply a matter of physical contact or even chemical reactions. As we discussed in chapter 3, according to Chinese medicine, we are surging with electromagnetic energy that travels through specific pathways, called meridians, to every corner of our body. We can exchange this energy with our partner through our touch. Our fingertips, our lips and tongues, and our genitals are the most powerful ways in which we can exchange this energy with each other.

When you touch your partner, focus on your hands and imagine loving energy flowing from your fingers into your partner's body. Remember, our chi, or energy, follows our mind. Touch is touch, but ecstatic, healing touch requires attention and love.

Touch is touch, but ecstatic, healing touch requires attention and love.

LIKE THE WEIGHT OF A FEATHER

Energetic and sensual touch is featherlight touch that simply grazes over the surface of your partner's skin, awakening the nerve endings and drawing energy to the area. In a massage, harder pressure will relax your partner's muscles, while light touch will awaken your partner's skin.

For sensually touching a woman, a man needs to remember that her sexual energy needs to be brought to her vagina from the extremities of her body.

For sensually touching a woman, a man needs to remember that her sexual energy must be brought to her genitals from her extremities. Time providing, he should start at her hands and feet and move along her legs and arms. Then he can start at her head and caress along her torso. Only after circling her genitals should he touch them directly. In the metaphors of the Tao, yin is like water and so it must fall down the mounds and folds of a woman's curvaceous body to the lowest point, her vagina. Water always settles in the lowest place.

For sensually touching a man, a woman needs to remember that his sexual energy needs to be brought out of his penis to the rest of his body.

For sensually touching a man, a woman needs to remember that his sexual energy needs to be brought out of his penis to the rest of his body. For this reason, she can start at his penis, touching it lightly but without focusing on direct stimulation. She does not want to stoke his fire but to keep it at a low burn. If he gets too excited, he will explode and ejaculate. By taking the sexual energy from a man's genitals, his partner can spread it out through his legs and arms, out to his hands and feet, and up to his torso and head. This will draw the energy away and allow him to have greater ejaculatory control and help him experience whole-body orgasms.

Of course, if he is having difficulty with an erection, the energy should be drawn *to* his penis. (Bear in mind, when a man lies on his back, gravity works against his maintaining an erection as the blood flows out. If maintaining an erection is an issue, it is best for the man not to lie on his back, so that gravity can draw blood to his penis, not away from it. Standing, sitting, kneeling, and lying over his partner are all better positions for helping a man to get an erection.)

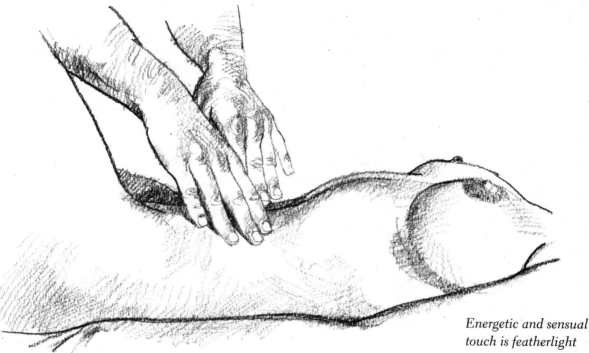

Energetic and sensual touch is featherlight and simply grazes over the surface of your partner's skin, awakening the nerve endings and drawing energy to the area.

Body Parts

In the West, we tend to think of people as machines and the parts of our body as separate, like the parts of a car. When touching your partner's body, it is important to remember that the energy meridians (channels) circulate throughout the body and that you are trying to awaken your partner's sexual energy and not just to stimulate a particular part of his or her body. Put differently, great pleasure can be generated by touching particular nerve endings on our hands and feet or nipples and genitals, but these nerves are connected through a complex web with the rest of the body. Try to maintain a holistic and energetic view of your partner's body even as you refine your skills for pleasuring individual parts. In Healing Love, every touch is part of harmonizing with each other; holding hands or pressing lips together is as important as intercourse.

While the suggestions below are based on ancient observation and modern study, they are of course just generalizations. You and your partner will have your own ways to please each other and your own preferences for how you like to be pleased. We recommend that you read these sections together and discuss your own unique sensitivities and desires.

In addition, every sexual encounter will be different. In a midday quickie, you may both be genitally focused, while a leisurely weekend evening may afford you the time to explore every inch of each other's erotic landscape. It is always best to have a few favorite songs memorized but to improvise like good jazz musicians.

Let's take it from the top, with a few pleasures not to be missed.

LIPS AND TONGUES

Most people begin instinctively with kissing, as they harmonize their desire and share their breath with their partner. Lips and tongues can offer almost endless pleasure as partners fuse their mouths together.

According to the Taoists, the lips and tongue are one of the main channels for exchanging energy, so they strongly recommended extended kissing and "French" kissing (which they discovered independently of the French). When you touch lips and tongues, send your partner your energy and drink in your partner's energy.

For the Taoists, saliva was considered a supreme elixir, a life-giving cocktail, but remember that both partners should agree on how much spit to swap. Many men like it wetter than many women. You can always ask your partner to kiss you as he or she likes to be kissed.

SCALP

The scalp is the crown of the body and also its energetic peak. You can help stimulate the top of your partner's head and draw energy here by scratching your partner's scalp as you would an itch or a kitty cat. From here you can start drawing the energy down the front channel of your partner's body by stroking or kissing down the front of his or her body.

EARS

According to Chinese medicine, the ears are filled with acupuncture points and are extremely sensitive to touch, tongues, and even breath.

SPINE

The spine is extremely sensitive along the neck and down to the tailbone. As we discussed earlier, the spine is a major channel for conducting energy from the genitals up to the brain, and, as you embrace, it will help your partner if you lightly stroke up the spine to help them draw the energy up.

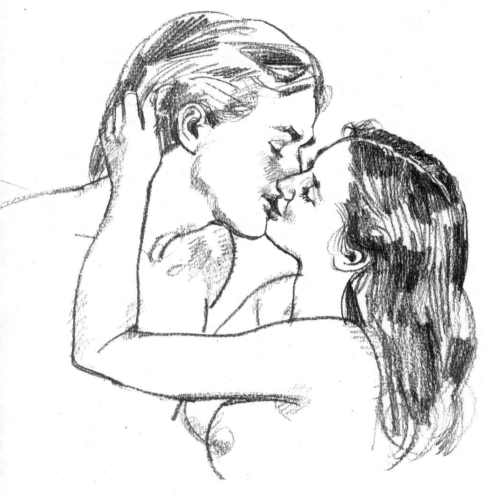

According to the Taoists, the lips and tongue are one of the main channels for exchanging energy.

HANDS AND FEET

Our hands and feet are some of our most sensitive and sexually exciting parts of our body. The size and shape of fingers and toes make them perfect for licking and sucking in ways that can drive your partner into gyrations of pleasure. Kissing and licking the palm of your partner's hand and wrist can be especially tantalizing.

ARMS AND LEGS

Arms and legs respond well to featherweight touching, and the inner thighs are especially responsive to sexual touch and licking as you move to your partner's genitals.

BREASTS, HERS AND HIS

Spiraling around the breast in increasingly smaller circles draws the energy to the nipple. Rubbing your thumb and finger together prior to touching your partner's nipples generates chi that can increase your partner's stimulation. Eventually, touch your partner's nipples between your thumbs and fingers and lightly roll the nipples between them. (You may wish to start with one at a time.)

While the nipples are certainly the most sensitive part of a woman's breast, most women enjoy having their entire breasts touched and massaged before their partner zeros in on their nipples.

Women differ greatly in the amount of stimulation they like and how hard they like their breasts to be fondled and their nipples squeezed. In general, the more aroused a woman becomes, the harder the stimulation she will find pleasurable, which is one reason that women often find they enjoy more intense nipple stimulation later during prolonged foreplay or intercourse.

Men's breasts and nipples are far less prominent and generally much less sensitive than women's. This has led to the mistaken belief that men's nipples are not sensitive. Many men find that their nipples are very sensitive and even get erect, while others need regular stimulation to awaken these nerve endings. Finally, some men never warm to nipple stimulation or would just prefer their partner move on to more sensitive spots.

As we mentioned above, the tongue is an extraordinary conduit of chi, and there is no better way to arouse your partner's nipples than with your tongue.

There is a triangle of arousal between nipples (for women and men) and genitals. Stimulating a woman's (or man's) nipples will often stimulate the genitals at the same time or at least start an itch below that demands to be scratched.

GENITALS, HERS

A woman's clitoris has the greatest concentration of nerve endings in the body, and it is because of this intense sensitivity that it must be touched with real care and real understanding. As with the nipples, the more engorged the clitoris is, the more intense stimulation will be enjoyable. Circling around the clitoris, as with the nipples, will draw energy to it and help prepare a woman's clitoris for direct stimulation. This circling is essential for stoking her fire and bringing her desire to a boil.

A man should generally begin by stroking or spiraling on the less sensitive base and sides of the clitoris. He can also roll the clitoris through the lips of the vagina. Then try gently stroking or spiraling on the hood before touching

In general, the more aroused a woman becomes, the harder the stimulation she will find pleasurable, which is one reason that women often find they enjoy more intense nipple stimulation later during prolonged foreplay or intercourse.

the extremely sensitive glans itself. For some women direct stimulation of the glans is always too intense, so a man needs to follow his partner's lead here (moans, pants, sweat, smiles, or verbal cues).

Clitoral stimulation is essential for most women to experience orgasm. Many women take longer to orgasm through intercourse because their clitoris is not being directly stimulated. Imagine a man trying to orgasm while just stroking the base of his penis or his testicles but not stimulating the head of his penis! If this were the case, many books might be written about the difficulty men have in reaching orgasm.

Repeatedly women have been shown to orgasm just as fast as men during self-pleasuring (and while stimulating their clitoris). The mistake that many couples make is assuming that a woman should not touch herself during sex or that the clitoris does not need to be stimulated during intercourse.

A man can learn a great deal about how a woman likes to have her clitoris stimulated if she is willing to show him. She can begin by touching herself

Clitoral stimulation is essential for most women to experience orgasm. Many women take longer to orgasm through intercourse because their clitoris is not being directly stimulated.

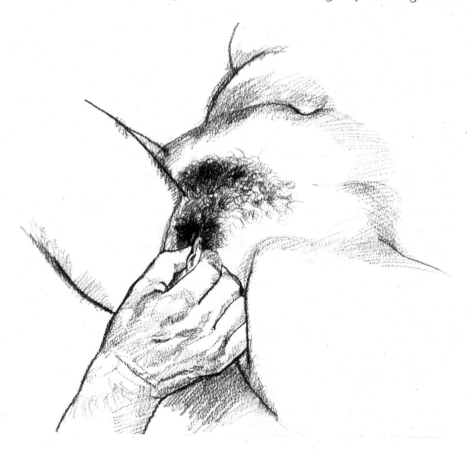

Rolling the clitoris between the lips of the vagina

and letting her partner rest his fingertips over hers and feel the place and pressure that she enjoys. Alternatively, she can rest her fingers on her partner's as she directs him to the place and pressure she wants. During intercourse, he (or she) can touch her clitoris and intensify her arousal and stimulation. Once couples learn this way of enhancing stimulation during intercourse, they will never have to worry about the woman's satisfaction or whether it was "good for her."

PLEASURING OURSELVES WHILE WITH OUR PARTNER

Many people feel ashamed of touching themselves in private let alone with their partner. They have been told that self-pleasuring is sinful or shameful, and the idea of touching themselves in front of their lover may sound shocking or embarrassing. It is difficult to transcend what is often years of social conditioning about masturbation. If you feel ashamed, the first thing you need to know is that you are not alone. The second thing you need to know is that shame about self-pleasuring is not natural. The puritanical view of sexuality is only one view of human sexuality. For Taoists, who see sexuality as an essential part of human health, masturbation is called solo cultivation and genital exercise. This exercise is seen as an essential part of cultivating our sexual and overall health.

Masturbation, or self-pleasuring, is also not something that is only for teenagers or singles. The American Medical Association in a book entitled *Human Sexuality* explained that masturbation is common among men and women of all ages, and women actually tend to masturbate more as they get older. One estimate suggests that 70 percent of all married men and women pleasure themselves.[3]

Many people feel that if their partner masturbates it somehow is a criticism of them or their desirability. Self-pleasuring does not take the place of partnered sex; rather, it can be a valuable complement. A sex study conducted by the University of Chicago found that people who are having sex regularly with a partner actually pleasure themselves more than people who are not.[4]

Even those who feel comfortable touching themselves in private often are reluctant to touch themselves in front of their partner. Often we feel vulnerable when we touch ourselves in front of our partner and show our desire. While this can be very frightening, true intimacy (sexual or any other) depends on vulnerability. If you can encourage and support each other to be vulnerable and reveal your desire in the bedroom, you are much more likely to show your vulnerability and open your hearts to each other in the rest of your relationship.

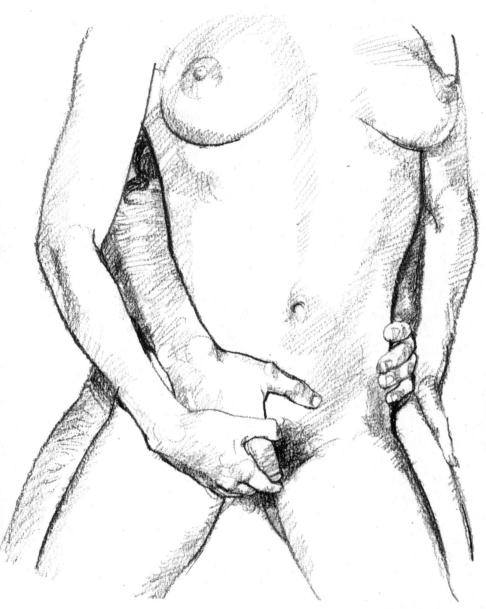

A woman can rest her fingers on her partner's as she directs him to the place and pressure she likes best.

Guiding your partner's hand to his or her own genitals during intercourse is one way to encourage them to reveal their desire. But don't push before they're ready if they resist. We cannot be forced to be vulnerable. Creating a loving, supporting, and intimate sexual and emotional relationship is the best way to help each other open up in the bedroom.

While the desire to please one's partner is a noble one, the truth is that everyone is responsible for his or her own orgasm. We can never give someone an orgasm for the very reason that orgasm takes place in our own brain.

Some people may feel threatened by their lover touching herself or himself during sex. They may feel that it is their role and responsibility to please their partner and feel uncomfortable when that role or responsibility is questioned. While the desire to please one's partner is a noble one, the truth is that everyone is responsible for his or her own orgasm. We can never give someone an orgasm for the very reason that orgasm takes place in our own brain.

FINGERING

When a man uses his fingers to enter his partner, he can explore her G spot and other sensitive spots with greater precision than he can with his penis. Before entering his partner, a man should linger at her vaginal lips, playing with them and her clitoris until she is very wet and engorged. The more lubricated and engorged she is, the more pleasurable his fingering will be.

If she is not completely lubricated, he can use saliva or oil on his finger as a lubricant or try oral sex (below), which brings its own natural lubrication. Besides saliva, natural oils or water-based lubricants are best. Never use Vaseline or scented oils or lotions, which can irritate the vagina. Remember that oils will break down latex and should not be used with condoms. Whatever you use, lubrication is important. If the woman is dry, a man's best-intentioned explorations will feel uncomfortable and often painful.

In addition to getting his partner wet, another reason to be slow to enter her is to build anticipation. As mentioned above, yin is slower than yang, and when a man can have a slow hand, he will bring his partner's desire to a rapid and eager boil. When he does enter her, she will be much more receptive to and desirous of his finger play. In addition, a woman's G spot (and other spots) will be much easier to find and much more sensitive as she approaches and even experiences orgasm.

THE A, B, C, AND G SPOTS

The G spot is an extremely pleasurable spot located about one and a half to two inches from the opening of the vagina on the upper wall (if the woman is lying on her back), just behind the pubic bone. If you are facing her vulva and you imagine a clock with the clitoris at twelve, the G spot is usually somewhere between eleven and one o-clock.

This spot is named after Dr. Ernest Gräfenberg, who was the first modern physician to describe this spot. Needless to say, women (and many men) have long known about this spot. The Taoists referred to it as the Black Pearl.

One of the best ways for a woman to be multi-orgasmic is to stimulate her clitoris during intercourse.

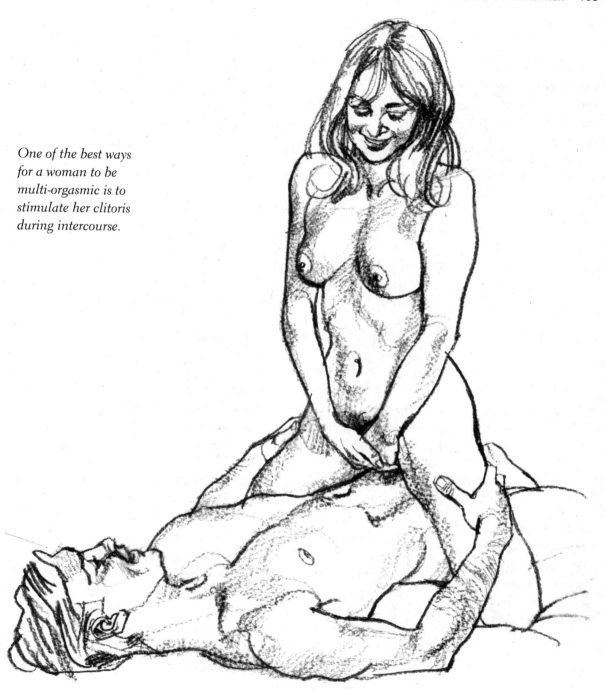

The G spot is an extremely pleasurable spot generally one-third to two-thirds of a finger from the opening of the vagina, just behind the pubic bone.

G SPOT

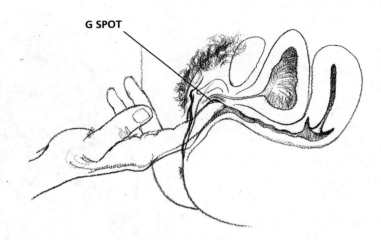

Whether all women have such a spot is still debated since some women have found it and others have not.

It is important to know a few G-spot basics before a man (or woman) starts exploring (see opposite).

The G spot is the most famous pleasure spot in a woman's vagina, but each woman has her own unique spots. The G spot, it seems, is simply erectile tissue that swells when it is stimulated. There are other sensitive spots that you can find. Most recently, X and Y spots have been discovered on the left and right sides of the G spot at about the same depth (about one and a half inches inside). Recent studies suggest that the clitoris, which was once believed to be a tiny structure in the body, is actually much larger and its nerves descend down the walls of the vagina.

The Taoists knew about the importance of stimulating this part of the vagina and described a ring of pleasure just inside the entrance of the vagina at about this same depth. It is for this reason that they emphasized the importance of shallow thrusting to the left and right and top and bottom (see "Real Screwing," p. 122).

Some women report very pleasurable spots at four and eight o'clock about halfway back along the vaginal wall. Other women report great pleasure in their cul-de-sac, often located above or (when lying on their back) below the cervix. As the man circles a finger or two around the vagina and explores, together you will find unique landmarks of pleasure.

As the man circles a finger or two around the vagina and explores, together you will find unique landmarks of pleasure.

Discovering the G Spot

- THE RIDGES OF PLEASURE: When a woman is not aroused, the G spot is difficult to find, although you can often feel some bumpy or ridged skin.

- POCKET CHANGE: When stimulated, it can swell to the size of a dime or larger.

- ONCE AROUSED: It is best to stimulate the G spot once a woman is already aroused and even approaching orgasm.

- BLADDER ALERT: Some women feel discomfort or even the urge to urinate when the G spot is stroked. This is quite normal and may be due to the G spot's proximity to a woman's urethra and bladder. If her partner lightens his touch and patiently stimulates this spot, the discomfort will generally turn to pleasure. If a woman is worried about this seeming need to urinate, she can empty her bladder first or try finding the spot herself in the privacy of the bathroom.

- TWO NERVES ARE BETTER THAN ONE: According to physiological studies, the vagina and the clitoris may have two different nerve pathways. A man can try stimulating his partner's G spot and clitoris at the same time, which can lead to extremely intense, explosive orgasms.

At the same time, it is important to remember that some women do not have one or more particular spots that are more sensitive than others. Women should not feel pressured to find spots, and if dedicated exploration does not reveal any hidden treasures, remember that the entire vagina is a treasure chest of pleasure for most women. In addition, during fingering (as with thrusting), a man should know that hitting a woman's cervix can be painful for some women. The cervix is usually deep inside a woman's vagina, but the location varies from woman to woman and even throughout her cycle. As a result, a slow and gentle hand is generally best.

THE ART OF FINGERING

- SMOOTH NAILS: Men should make sure their fingernails are short and smooth. Any sharp edges will be magnified in the hypersensitive skin of the clitoris and vagina.

- FROM BEHIND: While prostrating before a woman's vagina is fine for oral sex, it is actually a very awkward position for fingering. A man can try pleasuring her from behind, which will allow his fingers to approach her clitoris and vagina from the same angle from which she pleasures herself. (See illustration on p. 107.)

- A SLOW HAND: According to the Tao, entering a woman before she's ready is a major sexual faux pas. A man should hesitate and linger before entering a woman's vagina with his fingers (or his penis). The famous female sex adviser to the Yellow Emperor, Su Nu, explained that a woman will arch her back and raise her genitals toward her partner's fingers or penis when she is ready for him to enter her.

- SPIRAL: Use smooth circular movements around and over the clitoris. Avoid jerking or sharp movements. Remember how concentrated the nerve endings are here.

- BETWEEN HER LIPS: Try rubbing her clitoris between her vaginal lips and rubbing the lips themselves.

- G-SPOTTING: A man should make sure to investigate the G-spot area, which is generally on the top wall (when a woman lies on her back) about one and a half inches from the opening of her vagina (see illustration on p. 110). As he goes deeper into her vagina, he can continue to circle all sides of her vaginal canal. By raising her legs, a woman shortens her vaginal canal and allows her partner to explore the depths of her vagina.

- FOLLOW THE LEADER: If a woman is willing, the man can place his fingers on hers or have her place hers on his and see how she likes to please herself. Similarly, she can use the head of his penis to stimulate herself.

GENITALS, HIS

As we have mentioned, yang energy moves up from the genitals, and so with a man you may wish to draw energy from his genitals to the rest of his body. Lightly cup or caress his crotch and then spread this sexual energy throughout the rest of his body by lightly drawing your fingertips up the front or back of his torso. Most men experience their sexual energy and their orgasms almost exclusively in their crotch, so it is especially important to spread this life-giving energy to awaken and heal the rest of a man's body.

Because male sexuality ignites so quickly, many men want to move right to genital stimulation. While it is important to recognize this natural desire, a woman can help her man experience a much more satisfying and expanded orgasm if she takes some time to spread this sexual energy out from his genitals. Yang energy is explosive, and once awakened it wants to shoot out from a man's penis, causing him to ejaculate. By spreading this energy out, a woman can help a man control his ejaculation and eventually experience multiple whole-body orgasms.

Most men and woman gauge a man's arousal by the angle of his erection. Therefore, it is important to mention that when a woman spreads sexual energy throughout a man's body or stimulates different parts of his genitals, such as his testicles or perineum, he may not get an erection or may lose the one he has. This does not mean that he is not experiencing intense pleasure, but it can be a source of worry for one or both of you. Erections rise and fall with the flow of sexual energy and blood to the penis.

Also keep in mind that when a man lies on his back, gravity will draw blood away from his penis. In addition, men often find they lose their erection when they are being receptive. Taoists would explain that because yang is active, the man often loses some of his yang charge when he is being receptive. Many men find that when they become active again, taking the initiative and pleasuring their partner, they become erect very quickly.

The following stroking techniques do not require the man to have an erection to experience great pleasure. If the couple wants the man to get hard for penetration, she can stimulate the head of his penis more directly with her hands or mouth or he can take the initiative and become more active. Just as the clitoris is the most sensitive part of a woman's anatomy, the head of the penis is the most sensitive part of the man's. As we discuss in the next chapter, Taoists believed it is important to stimulate a man's entire genitals.

> **Yang energy is explosive, and once awakened it wants to shoot out from a man's penis, causing him to ejaculate. By spreading this energy out, a woman can help a man control his ejaculation and eventually experience multiple whole-body orgasms.**

THE ART OF STROKING

- LUBE HIM UP: Lubrication, whether oil or water based, is essential for stroking a man's genitals for any significant period of time. Oil is definitely the best for prolonged stimulation. While women eventually generate their own lubrication, men are completely dependent on outside lubrication. A lubricant will also intensify the sensation for him. Keep in mind, oil-based lubricants may weaken condoms, diaphragms, and cervical caps. If you are using these, choose a water-based lubricant.

- THE SPEED OF LIGHT: When most men self-pleasure, they stroke themselves very quickly and orgasm (generally ejaculate) as quickly as possible. This may be old, patterned behavior from masturbating secretly and worrying about getting caught. It is also the nature of yang to want activity, even frenzied activity. In Taoist sexuality, ejaculation is no longer the goal. Slowing down and enjoying the ride is preferable and can both intensify the eventual orgasm (or orgasms) and lead to greater ejaculatory control. Still, most men will want continued, intense pressure.

- SMOOTH STROKES: A woman should try not to jerk up and down but to keep her movements fluid as she strokes up and down on a man's penis. As with a hydraulic pump, the pressure and speed should not lessen as a woman switches direction.

- TEASING HIS TESTICLES: Most men's testicles are very sensitive, often too sensitive for more than delicate touch. You can stimulate his testicles by running your nails or fingertips over them. Some men enjoy gentle tugging on the skin of the scrotum (be careful not to squeeze their balls). They also sometimes enjoy having their testicles circled with the ring of your thumb and forefinger and gently tugged down. Making a snug ring stretches the skin of the testicles, making it very sensitive to light fingertip and nail stimulation (see illustration opposite).

- BETWEEN THE BALLS: On many men there is a very sensitive spot between their testicles following down from the underside of their penis. This spot can be quite pleasurable.

- THE MALE G SPOT: We tend to think that male sexuality is simply the penis and testicles. However, many men experience intense pleasure when having their prostate stimulated, and this deep pleasure has often been equated with a woman's G spot. The prostate can be stimulated externally through the perineum or internally through the anus (see illustration on p. 9).

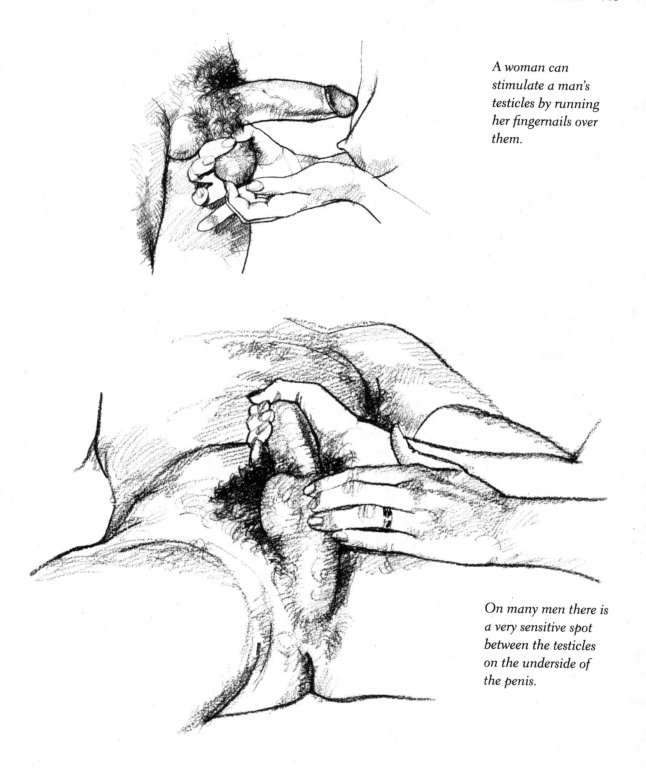

A woman can stimulate a man's testicles by running her fingernails over them.

On many men there is a very sensitive spot between the testicles on the underside of the penis.

Tongue Kung Fu: Oral Sex on Women

A recent survey concluded that most couples' relationships are happier when they're having oral sex.[5] A taboo for many modern couples until the 1960s, oral sex is now a regular part of many people's sexual repertoire, but most people do not rely on its harmonizing power enough.

For women, receiving oral sex, what the Taoists called Tongue Kung Fu, is the quickest way to have their desire brought to a boil and to become fully lubricated. While fingers can work wonders when sensitive and knowledgeable, they are too hard to really romance a woman's clitoris. A man's tongue and lips are more versatile and much better suited to pleasure her supremely sensitive clitoris and her vaginal lips.

It is worth mentioning that the porn industry has invented its own version of oral sex for the camera (in which a man rolls his head back and forth) that has little relationship to actual oral sex off camera. If you have ever watched oral sex in an adult movie, you will know how comical this depiction of the delicate and subtle art of cunnilingus is.

Mouth Kung Fu: Oral Sex on Men

For a man, receiving oral sex is so pleasurable that some men prefer it to intercourse. A woman's mouth and tongue allow her to pleasure her partner with pressure and precision that is rare during intercourse. (The PC exercises that we present in the woman's chapter and discuss again below will allow a woman to achieve similar skill and similar results with her vagina.) As with a woman, oral sex remains the quickest way to excite or resuscitate a man's desire when his heart is willing but his body is not quite ready.

Perhaps the best way to think of oral sex is as a hand job with the addition of the mouth's licking and sucking. In other words, while a woman's mouth is ideal for stimulating the head of a man's penis, her hands are often best suited for stimulating his shaft and his testicles. The combination of sucking and licking with stroking and fondling can certainly be exquisitely pleasurable.

For women, receiving oral sex, what the Taoists called Tongue Kung Fu, is the quickest way to have their desire brought to a boil and to become fully lubricated. While fingers can work wonders when sensitive and knowledgeable, they are too hard to really romance a woman's clitoris.

THE ART OF CUNNILINGUS

- **STRENGTHEN YOUR TONGUE:** Much of the success of "eating" a woman depends on the strength of a man's tongue. The Taoists realized this and developed practices to strengthen the muscles of the tongue so that this important muscle would be up to the task of pleasing a woman at length. The Taoist exercises are elaborate, but to begin with, a man can simply stick out and retract his tongue (like a snake) for a minute or two to strengthen it. (See *Taoist Secrets of Love: Cultivating Male Sexual Energy,* in the Resources section, for more advanced practices.)

- **ONLY SKIN DEEP:** Even a strong tongue cannot penetrate a woman as effectively as a finger or penis, so a man should focus his attention on her lips and clitoris.

- **LICKING:** A man can start at the bottom of the vagina and work his way up his partner's vaginal lips to her clitoris. At the clitoris, he can try rolling his tongue back and forth across her hood, spiraling in circles on her hood, and flicking up as he teases the clitoris itself.

- **SUCKING:** In addition to licking, the mouth is extremely good for sucking gently on a woman's lips and/or clitoris.

- **FINGER LICKING:** By eating his partner while inserting a finger into her vagina, a man can stimulate both her clitoris and her G spot or other spots inside her vagina. This very intense stimulation can send women into moans and multiple orgasms.

- **THE BERMUDA TRIANGLE:** There is a powerful triangle of arousal between most women's breasts and their vagina. By stimulating a woman's breasts while stimulating her clitoris, a man can intensify her pleasure greatly.

- **DRINKING:** The Taoists viewed a woman's vaginal waters as one of the great elixirs and encouraged men to drink in their partner's chi from her vagina, or what they called the Jade Chamber. Still, don't forget to leave enough lubricant (either her juices or your saliva) if planning coital locomotion.

- **EAT, EAT, EAT:** The Taoists were adamant about the value of oral sex for bringing a woman's waters to a rapid boil and strongly encouraged men to eat their partners until they begged for intercourse.

THE ART OF FELLATIO

- START SMALL: A woman can certainly take her partner in her mouth when he is small and not yet hard. This is an excellent way to raise his sexual energy if he is slow to get aroused or in later stages of lovemaking. It is perhaps the quickest way to help a man become erect (also see the Soft Entry technique, which the Taoists swore by, in chapter 8). For women who are hesitant to give their partners blow jobs or are intimidated by a hard penis, this is also a good place to start, since the flaccid penis is quite friendly and unintimidating.

- NO BLOWING IN THE WIND: Most women know, of course, that there is no blowing in a blow job. The job to be done almost exclusively involves licking and sucking. In fact, alternating between licking and sucking is generally a good idea.

- LICKING: For licking, the underside of the head of the penis, or frenulum, is generally the most sensitive, although a man's partner should explore his genitals from stem to stern. Don't forget to lick and flick his testicles. You can also stimulate his "male G spot" (see above) by pressing and massaging your tongue between his testicles at the base of his penis.

- SUCKING: The most sensitive spot for sucking is also the head of a man's penis, and sucking and licking this area can work wonders. Of course, sucking can also involve a deeper enveloping of a man's penis with your mouth. This deeper method feels good along the shaft of the penis, and the pressure of the back of the mouth feels extremely good on the sensitive head. When combined with a sucking action, this is the closest, some men swear, that they come to experiencing heaven on earth. As women become more experienced, they can often take their partner deeper into their mouth and even into their throat. This requires quite a bit of practice, and it is generally best if the woman controls the rhythm and depth of penetration.

- BYPASSING THE GAG REFLEX: Many women worry that they will gag if they take their partner deep into their mouth or throat. The woman can generally control the depth by using her jaw muscle and clamping down on his penis (preferably using her lips rather than her teeth, although if he's not listening teeth can get his attention). She can also use her hands to control the depth, and if her hands are on his penis, as we strongly recommend they should be (see below), she is certainly in the driver's seat. When the man is lying on his back, the woman has the most control of the situation. Many men love to be on top or to thrust into their partner's mouth, which often feels most like intercourse. This, however, takes good communication and coordination to make sure that he does not enter too deeply.

- LIPS AND TEETH: While an occasional nip or teasing bite on the head of the penis can be highly arousing, lips are generally more conducive to oral sex than teeth, especially for sucking and stroking his penis with your mouth.

- TO SWALLOW OR NOT TO SWALLOW: That is the question. Most women have had to come to their own decision about whether they want to swallow their partner's semen. For many women this concerns intimacy as well as taste and aesthetics. Some women will swallow one partner's ejaculate and not another's or at certain times and not others. With this said, it is worth mentioning that just as the taste and smell of a woman's vaginal juices change with her cycle and her diet, so too do the taste and smell of a man's semen. As a man learns to separate orgasm from ejaculation, this may no longer be the question.

- SWALLOWING CHI: While the Taoists saw swallowing semen as a way for a woman to receive energy from her partner, they did not strongly recommend it, given their encouragement that men experience orgasm without ejaculating. They also felt that most men lose more energy by ejaculating than their partner can possibly absorb. Just as a man can receive his partner's energy from cunnilingus, a woman can receive her partner's energy from fellatio without her partner ejaculating.

- KEEPING COOL: As we discuss in the following chapters, the Taoists recommended placing similar body parts together (mouth to mouth, genitals to genitals) for harmonizing and relaxing and placing dissimilar body parts together (such as mouth to genitals) for stimulating and exciting. In addition, when a man makes love his yang energy is cooled by his partner's yin, which can help him control his ejaculation.

Because oral sex is highly arousing without the cooling yin influence of intercourse, most men have a difficult time not ejaculating. Assuming a man does not want to ejaculate, it may be best for a woman to get her partner hot with oral sex but not try to bring him to orgasm. Alternatively, as her partner becomes more experienced at separating orgasm from ejaculation, he can control the rhythm or even help stimulate himself as he is getting close to the point of no return. A man's stroking himself while he receives oral sex can be extremely arousing to both partners but can also give the man better control of his arousal rate.

Shallow and Deep

When intercourse is shown in the media, it is almost always the mattress-spring-squeaking, in-and-out kind that leads to fast ejaculation and little satisfaction for either partner. The Taoists realized that proper thrusting is essential for pleasure during lovemaking, ejaculatory control, and overall sexual health. They strongly encouraged that couples wait until the woman is highly aroused before intercourse. In the parlance of the Taoists, a couple needs to wait until the woman's pot is boiling before the man puts his carrot and peas in. Otherwise, they will have soggy sex and his carrot will quickly be limp.

When most people think of intercourse, they think of being "in" or "out." For the Taoists, who mapped the pleasure points and reflexology points of the penis and vagina, there were many different depths and directions for the man to thrust and pleasure himself and, even more important, his partner. As explained in the next chapter, these points correspond with the organs and glands of the body, which are energized and healed by rubbing.

While you should experiment with various depths and directions, for the purposes of simplicity it is helpful to think of three basic thrusts: shallow thrusts, long deep thrusts, and short deep thrusts (see illustration on p. 122).

Finding a Rhythm That Works for Both of You

. The Taoists strongly recommended that men (or women, if they are on top) vary the type of thrusts they use. When used together, the deep thrusts push the air out of the woman's vagina and create a vacuum that can be intensified by using the shallow thrusts. As long as the penis does not come out completely, the vacuum effect is maintained.

The most important thing is to find a regular rhythm that you enjoy and then innovate and experiment with depth, direction, and speed.

The Taoists recommended using nine shallow thrusts and one long deep thrust as a basic rhythm or nine short deep thrusts and one long deep thrust. The long deep thrusts, although highly pleasurable, can make it hard for a man to control his ejaculation, while the short deep thrusts are deeply satisfying to the woman while not being overly stimulating to the man. As a man learns greater ejaculatory control and becomes multi-orgasmic, the thrusting ratio can be lessened to six or even three shallow or short deep and then one long deep. The most important thing is to find a regular rhythm that you enjoy and then innovate and experiment with depth, direction, and speed.

Finding the Way

Three Thrusts

- SHALLOW THRUSTS: These stimulate the highly sensitive first two inches of a woman's vagina and, depending on the position, her G spot.

- *LONG* DEEP THRUSTS: These are deep thrusts in which the man draws back almost to the entrance of the woman's vagina between thrusts. These are the thrusts that are depicted in the media and in pornography. They are highly stimulating for both partners, as the man pushes and pulls the head of his penis along the whole length of his partner's vagina.

- *SHORT* DEEP THRUSTS: These are deep thrusts in which the man stays deep in the woman and thrusts forward and back. This stimulates her clitoris (with the pressure from his pubic bone) and the back of her vagina while not stimulating the head of his penis nearly as much.

Of course, if the man is having difficulty getting or maintaining an erection, the long deep thrusts are extremely good for resolving this problem. Taoists realize that at some time or another every man has difficulty having an erection when he wants one. This is what sex therapists call "situational impotence." In these "situations," Taoists feel it is essential for a man to know the Soft Entry technique (see chapter 8). In ordinary ejaculatory sex, men enter hard and exit soft. In the Tao way, a man can enter hard or soft and exit hard.

The short deep thrust, which in *The Multi-Orgasmic Man* we called the "up down deep thrust," is excellent for ejaculatory control and to use when the woman is reaching orgasm and wants her man's penis deep inside her. With this thrust, the man can oblige her without risk of being pulled over the ejaculatory cliff.

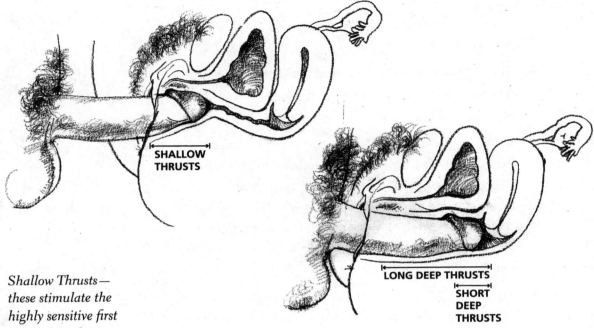

*Shallow Thrusts—
these stimulate the
highly sensitive first
two inches of a
woman's vagina.*

*Deep Thrusts—these
fill a woman fully. In
long deep thrusts, the
man draws back
almost to the entrance
and rubs the head of
his penis against the
whole length of the
vagina. In short deep
thrusts the man stays
deep inside the
woman and thrusts
forward, drawing back
only slightly.*

Depth, Direction, and Speed

The Taoists taught couples to vary the direction and speed of the thrust in addition to varying depth. The following descriptions are addressed to the man, but they also can be adapted fruitfully by the woman when she is on top. Remember, poetry and variety are wonderful, but the most important part of lovemaking is to be in your body, not your head. Be careful you don't get overly concerned with the type of thrust and lose the pleasure of the thrust itself.

Real Screwing

While we describe intercourse in English as "screwing," many couples don't actually screw each other; that is, they don't rotate their sacrum in circles. While the term itself has been seen as somewhat vulgar, the results when actually done are sublime. Instead of simply thrusting forward and pulling back, you can "screw" your hips or, ideally, your sacrum in half circles, first on one side and then on the other.

More experienced lovers the world over have discovered the importance of using one's pelvis (ideally sacrum) during lovemaking. The hips are good,

Finding the Way

Nine Taoist Thrusts

The following description is from the seventh-century physician Li Tung-hsuan Tzu, who suggested thrusts of varying depths, directions, and speeds.

1. Strike left and right as a brave general breaking through the enemy's ranks. [The battle-of-the-sexes imagery was not completely absent from Taoist sexuality.]
2. Rise and suddenly plunge like a wild horse bucking through a mountain stream.
3. Push and pull out like a flock of seagulls playing on the waves.
4. Use deep thrusts and shallow teasing strokes, like a sparrow plucking pieces of rice.
5. Make shallow and then deeper thrusts in steady succession [to the left and right], like a large stone sinking into the sea.
6. Push in slowly as a snake entering its hole.
7. Charge quickly like a frightened mouse running into its hole.
8. Hover and then strike like an eagle catching an elusive hare.
9. Rise up and then plunge down low like a great sailboat in a wild wind.

but, according to the Tao, it is the sacrum that really controls the penis for the man. To find your sacrum, place the palm of your hand at the base of your spine with the tip of your longest finger in the valley between your buttocks. Underneath your palm is your sacrum. This screwing can keep you connected in pleasure for a long time. In the language of the Tao, a nail (going in straight) comes out easily, but a screw (circling) stays in for a long time.

Instead of simply thrusting forward and pulling back, you can "screw" your hips or, ideally, your sacrum in half circles, first on one side and then on the other.

Rotating Your Sacrum

At first your rotations will probably come from your hips and pelvis, since, unless you do a lot of Latin or African dance, you are probably not accustomed to rotating your sacrum. Give it time, but eventually you will be able to spiral, to "screw," with subtle movements of your sacrum. To isolate your sacrum, you can put one hand on your pubis and one hand on your sacrum (just below your spine between your buttocks). Now try to spiral left and right. Next, try tilting your pubis up as you push your tailbone (the base of your sacrum) forward (curving your back out slightly), and then try tilting your penis down as you push your tailbone back (arching your spine slightly). Once you've isolated your sacrum, you can really screw.

Getting Really Hot

As the man gets highly aroused and close to the point of ejaculation, he and his partner can encourage him to slow down (stop if necessary) and do the deep breathing and PC muscle contractions to hold off ejaculation. While this momentary pause may seem like a nuisance at first, it will soon be forgotten as his ejaculatory control and eventual multiple orgasms allow far longer and more satisfying lovemaking. As the man masters his breathing and PC muscle, these pauses will be less frequent and less noticeable. In addition, both partners can circulate energy away from their genitals and through their bodies as we described in the previous chapter.

The multiple orgasms will increase the man's energy greatly, and not ejaculating will allow him to remain more yang. He will desire his partner more and become aroused more quickly. Of course, if the man has a lot of yang energy and either partner just wants to go to sleep, he can always ejaculate. In addition, both partners can circulate energy away from their genitals and through their bodies.

In the next chapter, we also discuss various practices and positions for profound health as well as pleasure, but first let us summarize the practices we have been discussing above.

THE ART OF INTERCOURSE

- LINGERING: The Taoists strongly recommended that a couple wait until the woman is extremely wet and yearning for intercourse. Entering too early, they believed, does not allow the sexual energy to enter her genitals and to make the lovemaking most healing and energizing. We also know that having intercourse too soon does not allow time for the woman to become fully engorged and results in her genitals being less sensitive and less stimulated by penetration. Still, lingering does not rule out quickies; it simply means that the man must pay special attention to making sure that his partner is highly aroused, lubricated, and eager for intercourse. His mouth can expedite this state of things greatly.

- SHALLOW AND DEEP: Varying the depth of thrusts is one of the most important Taoist techniques. The Taoists knew that by varying the depth a couple can stimulate different parts of the penis and vagina. The Taoists also recommended varying shallow and deep thrusts as a way of allowing the man to control his ejaculation so he can be multi-orgasmic and help his partner to be also. The long deep thrusts are often very stimulating to the man as he stimulates the head of his penis along the whole length of his partner's vagina and enters into her tight cul-de-sac. Shallow thrusts can often be less intense for him while still quite stimulating for her.

- SHORT DEEP THRUSTS: The real Taoist secret of male ejaculatory control and female satisfaction during intercourse is the short deep thrust. Here, the man remains deep inside his partner and thrusts forward and back, pressing both against her deep vaginal walls with his penis and against her clitoris with his pubic bone. By not moving in and out very much, the man does not highly stimulate himself but deeply pleasures his partner. This is an extremely good thrust when the man is close to ejaculating and when his partner is eager for deep thrusting.

- VACUUM SEALED: A couple can also use deep and then shallow thrusts to create an intense vacuum that is especially stimulating for the woman. When a man finally enters a woman fully with a deep thrust, his penis pushes out all of the air in her vagina. By then making a series of shallow thrusts without breaking the seal (that is, pulling out completely), he creates a vacuum that can be intensely pleasurable.

- DANCING IN THE SHEETS: The Taoists recommended that a couple, and especially a man, rotate the hips (ideally, the sacrum) to really "screw." Screwing allows the man to stimulate all the walls of a woman's vagina. The rocking of the hips or sacrum is also excellent for channeling the energy up the spine.

CHAPTER 5

Sexual Healing

In this chapter you will discover:

- The Power of Sex to Heal Us and Keep Us Young
- The Art of Sexual Healing
- The Reflexology Points on the Genitals
- The Art of Taoist Genital Massage
- Sexual Positions for Harmonizing and Healing
- How to Circulate Healing Sexual Energy During Lovemaking
- The Effects of Ejaculation on a Man's Energy and Health
- How to Strengthen Your Sex Organs
- How Healing Love Can Help You Have Safer Sex

Most modern people have come to think that sex is exclusively for pleasure and/or procreation. Public discussions about sex are generally debates over pleasure and perversion: with whom you can and cannot have sex, what you can and cannot do, when you can and cannot do it. This rather narrow focus misses the larger value of sex and sexual energy in our lives. For Taoists, sex is as much about health as it is about either pleasure or procreation. Healing Love developed out of the Chinese medical tradition, and Taoists have long known that sexuality is as important to our overall well-being as nutrition or exercise. Orgasm is not simply a momentary release but a life-giving part of our overall health and longevity.

Orgasm is not simply a momentary release but a life-giving part of our overall health and longevity.

The Fountain of Youth

According to the Taoists, it is essential for us to feel the arousal of our sexual energy and orgasm as often as possible—ideally, every day. (As should be obvious by now, for men the Taoists were talking about orgasm without ejaculation.) During arousal and orgasm our body releases sexual hormones that for the Taoists are literally the fountain of youth. Modern medical research is also discovering the enormous health benefits that sex and orgasm can offer.

In one recent study breast cancer survivors who experienced orgasms through lovemaking or self-pleasuring recovered more quickly than those who did not.[1] Perhaps the most startling research suggests that sex and especially orgasm may even prolong our lives. The *British Medical Journal* reported that the more orgasms men in their study had the less likely they were to die. Of the 918 men between the ages of 45 and 59, those who had frequent orgasms, defined as twice a week or more, had a 50 percent lower mortality rate than those men who had infrequent orgasms, defined as less than one per month. This lower mortality rate was true for death from all causes as well as death from coronary heart disease, the most common killer in the United States. In addition, there was a "dose-response relation"—the more often a man had sex, the lower his chance was of dying.[2]

Chemically, we now know that the beneficial hormone oxytocin, which we discussed in the last chapter, and PEA, which has been called the molecule of love and is an amphetamine–like upper, both peak at orgasm.[3] Regular sex also increases the amount of testosterone in both men's and women's bodies, and testosterone both improves thinking and functions as an antidepressant.

In addition, exercise experts are starting to believe that even relatively brief physical exercise can generate major aerobic benefits for the body and the immune system. Therefore, even nonmarathon sex can have substantial physical benefits for your whole body.

For thousands of years Westerners have been searching for the legendary fountain of youth. This search took them around the world. What Taoists have always known is that the fountain of youth is in our very own bedroom.

What Taoists have always known is that the fountain of youth is in our very own bedroom.

When Sparks Fly: Sexual Energy Healing

The Taoists also believed that the value of Healing Love goes beyond the mere physical or biochemical. In Chinese medicine, health benefits occur as healing energy is channeled through the body. As writer Daniel Reid points out,

According to the Tao, a brief burst of explosive energy occurs when a man or woman reaches orgasm. Western science has already established that, at the point of sexual orgasm, human brain wave patterns alter radically, literally putting the person into an "altered state of consciousness." Profound physiological and electrical changes occur throughout the system during orgasm, and a burst of energy is indeed emitted.[4]

Through practicing Healing Love, you and your partner can learn to circulate this healing energy within your own body and to channel it to each other.

Circulating multi-orgasmic energy from your genitals to your head and then down to your abdomen, as described in chapter 3, has many health benefits. This multi-orgasmic energy, which can last as long as fourteen hours after lovemaking, nourishes your body and charges your brain.

Even before hearing about the hormonal and energetic health benefits of sex, you probably have intuitively known about how sex can make you feel better physically as well as psychologically. According to the Tao, this is not just because it *feels* good to you but also because it *is* good for you.

You have probably noticed that sometimes after lovemaking you feel better and more energized than at other times. Just as we can choose to eat healthier foods, Taoists believe we can choose to have healthier sex. There are several ways to make your lovemaking most healing.

THE ART OF SEXUAL HEALING

- LOVE IS HEALING: The emotions we bring to sex make a big difference in how healing it is for us and for our partner. If our heart is filled with love, it is much easier to circulate and transmit healing energy to our partner. If we bring negative emotions such as anger or frustration to our lovemaking, we are unable to circulate healing energy or to transmit it to our partner.

- LIMIT EJACULATIONS: As we have mentioned, the Taoists noticed the depletion that generally accompanies ejaculation and therefore recommended that as men get older they limit the number of times they ejaculate. They also encouraged men to limit ejaculation when sick or tired. Because they taught men to separate orgasm from ejaculation, men could experience multiple orgasms even without ejaculating.

- MULTIPLY ORGASMS: As couples multiply their orgasms, they not only multiply their pleasure; they also multiply their healing energy. If a man has several orgasms before ejaculating, he will lose less sexual energy should he ejaculate (see below).

- CIRCULATE ENERGY: The more energy an individual is able to circulate (see chapter 3) or a couple is able to exchange (see chapter 7), the more healing the lovemaking will be. First, you and your partner should try to circulate the energy in your own body, and eventually you can exchange energy with each other.

- HEALING PRACTICES: The Taoists encouraged couples to use healing practices like genital massage (see below) and healing positions to intensify the healing of their lovemaking. Use these practices as you please and as you need.

- TAKE YOUR TIME: According to the Tao, for lovemaking to be most healing, couples should arouse each other for at least a half hour with hugging, kissing, touching, and foreplay and then have multi-orgasmic intercourse for another half hour.

Mapping Your Genitals

Each part of the genitals corresponds with another part of the body. Through manual stimulation, oral sex, and intercourse, the entire body is stimulated and revitalized.

The Taoists discovered that, just as there are reflexology points on the foot that correspond with the rest of the body, each part of the genitals corresponds with another part of the body. Through manual stimulation, oral sex, and intercourse, the entire body is stimulated and revitalized. The healing benefits are considered very important, and for this reason the Taoists encouraged lovers to stimulate the entire penis and the entire vagina, especially the shaft of the man's penis and the entrance to the woman's vagina.

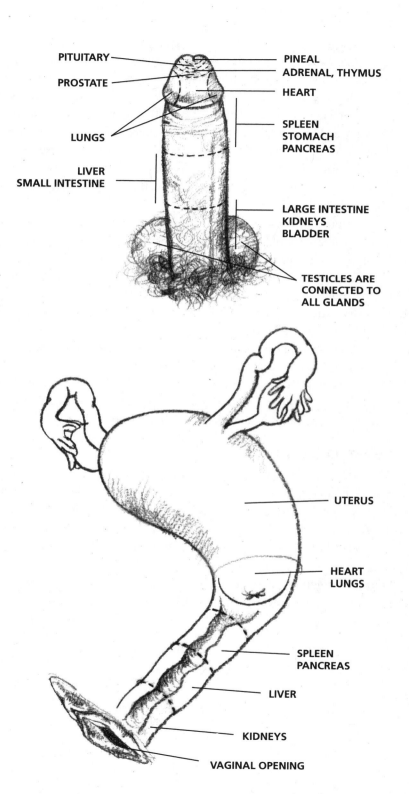

PITUITARY

PROSTATE

LUNGS

LIVER
SMALL INTESTINE

PINEAL
ADRENAL, THYMUS

HEART

SPLEEN
STOMACH
PANCREAS

LARGE INTESTINE
KIDNEYS
BLADDER

TESTICLES ARE
CONNECTED TO
ALL GLANDS

*Penis Reflexology—
each part of the penis
corresponds with
another part of a
man's body.*

UTERUS

HEART
LUNGS

SPLEEN
PANCREAS

LIVER

KIDNEYS

VAGINAL OPENING

*Vagina Reflexology—
each part of the
vagina corresponds
with another part of a
woman's body.*

In Healing Love, we try to stimulate these organ reflexology points on the shaft of the man's penis and the walls of the woman's vagina. The Taoists believed that the reflexology points are stronger on the sex organs than on the feet or hands and even more powerful than the acupuncture points on the ears and nose. The genitals connect directly to our internal organs, so you can directly stimulate an organ that is weak and in need of healing. Also, the Taoists recommended allowing the sexual energy to rise to individual organs for strengthening and healing the organ as well as for experiencing a more intense whole-body orgasm.

As we discuss below, in Exercise 18: Around the World in One Night, when the woman is able to squeeze around the shaft of the man's penis (avoiding too much stimulation of the head), the couple can become very highly aroused without the man's ejaculating. Once a couple understand the reflexology points of the genitals, they can experience not only genital pleasure but also extremely energizing "organ orgasms" that can last for up to ten hours. "Organ orgasms" were considered one of the great secrets of healing love. For a step-by-step discussion, please see Mantak and Maneewan Chia's book *Healing Love Through the Tao* (see Resources).

This concern with stimulating the entire penis and vagina also led the Taoists to discover many sexual positions that are both highly pleasurable and extremely healing. But first let us begin with our trusty hands.

TAOIST VAGINAL MASSAGE

While the goal of fingering (see previous chapter) is to heat a woman's passion to the boiling point or beyond, Taoist vaginal massage is different. Like a good body rub, Taoist vaginal massage is more interested in health than in heat. While not focused on passion, it still leads to great pleasure and is very good for exploring a woman's genital hot spots for future fingering or intercourse.

During the genital massage, a woman can circulate her sexual energy, which will bring pleasure and healing to the rest of her body.

THE ART OF TAOIST VAGINAL MASSAGE

- GET WET: Even more than fingering, genital massage requires lots of lubrication. A woman's own natural lubricant is best, but it is better to err in the direction of too much rather than too little lubrication.

- ENGORGED: The more engorged a woman is, the more sensitive her vagina will be. For this reason, her partner may wish to wait until later in lovemaking before giving her a genital rub.

- LIPS: A woman's partner can massage her lips and draw them away from her vagina (below, left). He can also try rubbing them together.

- ENTERING THE JADE CHAMBER: By inserting a finger or two into her vagina, a woman's partner can try stimulating different parts of her vaginal canal, which the Taoists affectionately called the Jade Chamber. Her partner should try circling a finger or two around her vagina, making sure to touch the top, bottom, and side walls (below, right). When he strikes a golden spot, obviously he can linger and explore. Remember, however, that the point of vaginal massage is not bringing your partner to orgasm. Keeping her aroused but not peaking is the goal.

- HEALING: The reflexology diagram on p. 131 shows the relationship the Taoists found between vaginal trigger points and the rest of a woman's body. Massaging these different rings, the Taoists believed, can bring health and healing to the corresponding parts of the body.

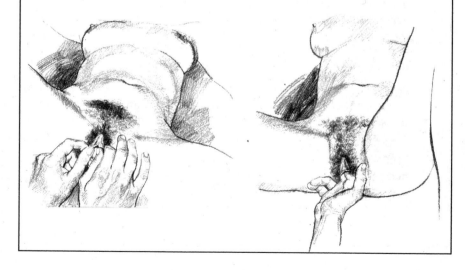

TAOIST PENIS MASSAGE

As with vaginal massage, penis massage is more about health than heat, more like a massage than masturbation. Still the techniques, skills, and sensitivities that are learned during massage can be applied whenever a woman is sexually stimulating her man.

Until a man learns to become multi-orgasmic, it is essential that his partner not push him over the ejaculatory edge. On an arousal scale of 1 to 10, if ejaculation is a 10 and orgasm is a 9.8, then the goal of genital massage is generally to keep a man simmering between a 7.0 and a 9.0. Once a man becomes multi-orgasmic, and with good verbal or bodily communication, his partner can take him up to orgasm and back down many times. But again, the goal is a pleasurable and healing massage more than scoring orgasms.

During the massage, the man can circulate his sexual energy throughout his body, which will help control his arousal and bring pleasure and healing to the rest of his body. If a man gets too hot, it is difficult for him to circulate his sexual energy, which is another reason why it is best to keep him on a low simmer.

THE ART OF TAOIST PENIS MASSAGE

- LUBE HIM UP: As with traditional hand jobs, lubrication is essential.

- ERECTION ALERT: A man does not need to be fully erect to receive a genital massage, and in fact most men's erections will wax and wane depending on the intensity of the stimulation. In addition, the fact that the man is lying on his back often means that gravity is working against his erection and will draw blood away from his penis. He may be experiencing intense pleasure whether or not he is erect.

- PRESSURE: The amount of pressure a woman uses is important. If the pressure of her hand on his penis is too much or too little it will decrease the sensation. As with any massage, experiment with the right amount of pressure.

- STROKES: There are many traditional genital massage strokes, and the number of strokes you use is limited only by your imagination. A marvelous video by Joe Kramer demonstrates several of them (see Resources). On the opposite page are some that you might not want to miss.

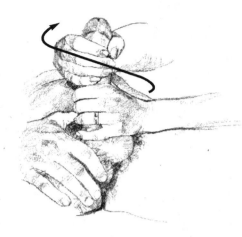

The corkscrew is a spiraled stroke up and down the shaft of the penis.

The underside of the head of the penis (called the frenulum) is perhaps the most sensitive part of the man's genitals. A man's partner can rub her thumbs up along the underside of the head one thumb at a time.

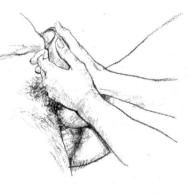

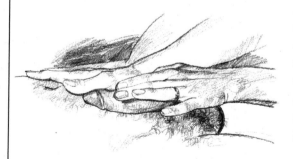

By rubbing the penis up along the stomach, his partner can both massage the sensitive underside of the penis and help him to spread sexual energy through his body.

Healing Positions

The Taoists believed that love expressed through sexuality is the most powerful medicine, and they called sex the "human herb." A Taoist physician would frequently prescribe several weeks of lovemaking in a specific position for a particular ailment.

We will discuss a number of healing positions below, but first we would like to give you some general guidelines for making all lovemaking more healing and satisfying.

The Taoists believed that love expressed through sexuality is the most powerful medicine, and they called sex the "human herb." A Taoist physician would frequently prescribe several weeks of lovemaking in a specific position for a particular ailment.

Finding the Way

Harmonizing and Healing

- HARMONIZING: For harmonizing and relaxing with each other, place similar body parts together: lips to lips, hands to hands, and genitals to genitals.

- STIMULATING: For stimulating and exciting each other, place dissimilar body parts together: lips to ear, mouth to genitals, genitals to anus.

- SWITCHING: When a man feels the urge to ejaculate, the couple should switch positions, which will switch the stimulation on his penis and allow him to control his ejaculation more easily. By the man's not ejaculating too soon, the couple will have time to generate more healing energy.

- HEALING: For healing each other, remember that the person who moves (generally the person on top) gives more energy to the other partner. In other words, if your partner is feeling tired, has little energy, or is not feeling well, you can give him or her energy by being on top and being more active during lovemaking. The person underneath can move as well to complement the movement of the person on top.

In the West, we tend to think that the person on top is the more powerful or dominant one. How different is the Taoist understanding, where the person on top (who is generally more active) is able to heal and give to the one underneath (who is generally more receptive).

The following are four basic positions from which all other positions are created. While the search for new positions is fun and can help stimulate various parts of our genitals, the most important factor in satisfying lovemaking is the quality of the connection, not the novelty of the position.

MAN ON TOP

In this position, which the missionaries made famous (and obligatory), the man lies on top of the woman, supporting himself on his hands or elbows.

This position is extremely good for harmonizing, since similar body parts are touching. In this position you can look into each other's eyes and kiss passionately. Both the eyes and the tongue are major conduits of healing energy.

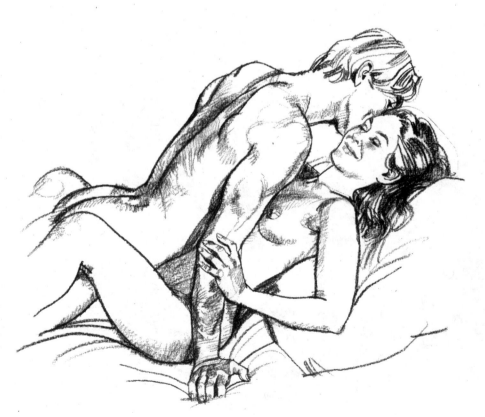

This position, which the missionaries made famous, is extremely good for harmonizing, since similar body parts are touching.

One major disadvantage of this position is that the woman's G spot is usually entirely bypassed as the man's penis presses against the back wall of her vagina. The man can address this problem by tilting his sacrum and pointing his penis up, or the woman can place a pillow under her buttocks, which has the same effect of changing the angle to press against the front wall of her vagina. Instead of a pillow, the woman can also rest her legs on the man's arms or shoulders.

When a woman raises her legs, she deepens the penetration: the higher her legs, the deeper the penetration. This can increase pleasure for both partners and is especially helpful if the female partner has a relatively large vagina or if the male partner has a relatively small penis.

Be aware that with deeper penetration the man is more likely to hit his partner's cervix, which for some women can be painful. When initiating this position, have the man enter slowly until a comfortable thrusting angle is found.

When the woman raises her legs, she deepens the penetration of her vagina—the higher the legs, the deeper the penetration

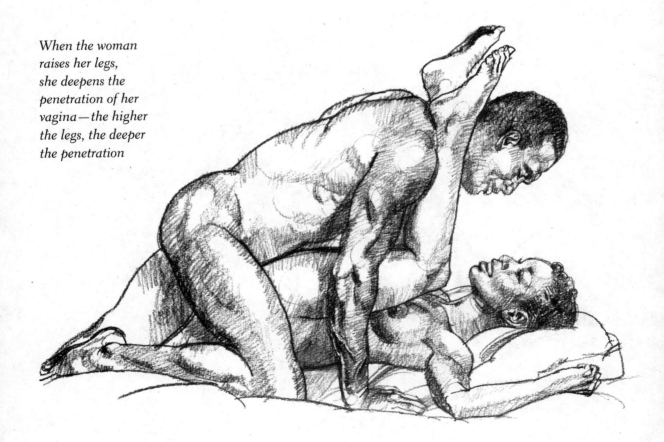

According to the Tao, the man-on-top position is often a good position in which to begin lovemaking. Because women are like water and men are like fire, this position allows the man to be active and to share his energy and heat with his partner. He can stoke the embers of his partner's desire. When the woman's desire is boiling over and risks quenching the man's fire (literally causing him to ejaculate), you may wish to switch positions and have the woman on top.

WOMAN ON TOP

In the woman-on-top positions, the man is lying on his back and the woman straddles him. Many men find that this is the easiest position in which to have multiple orgasms. In this position, the man can relax his pelvic muscles and pay close attention to his arousal rate. As he approaches the point of no return, he can squeeze his PC muscle. Gravity also helps draw energy away from the penis and allows the man to focus on channeling his energy up his spine.

Many men find that this is the easiest position in which to have multiple orgasms. In this position, the man can relax his pelvic muscles and pay close attention to his arousal rate.

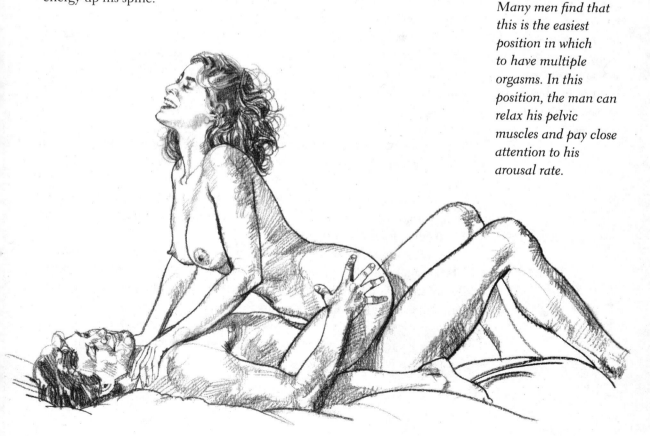

In this position, the man needs to be able to communicate when he is close to ejaculating and the woman needs to be willing to stop briefly before he reaches the point of no return. While this momentary interruption may seem irritating to the woman at first, it allows the man to control his ejaculation and to prolong lovemaking greatly, leading to far greater pleasure for her and for her partner. As the man becomes more skillful, these pauses will become fewer and will eventually become part of the natural ebb and flow of lovemaking. For the same reasons that this position makes it easier for a man to avoid ejaculating, it makes it more difficult for men with erection problems or less sexual energy to maintain an erection.

In this position, the woman can direct the head of her partner's penis to the most sensitive parts of her vagina, including her G spot, which is one reason that for many women this is also the easiest position in which to have (multiple) orgasms. In this position, the woman can also keep the head of her partner's penis in the often very sensitive outer two inches of her vagina.

This position also allows the man's hands to be free to stimulate the woman's clitoris, which can enhance her pleasure. The woman can also use her own hands to stimulate her clitoris, which together with the vaginal thrusting greatly increases the likelihood that she will experience multiple orgasms. Alternatively, the woman can press her clitoris against her partner's pubic bone during deep penetration. While the woman controls the thrusting and clitoral stimulation, the man can use his free hands to caress his partner's breasts and gently roll her nipples between his fingers.

If the woman leans forward or the man props his back and head up on a pillow, he can also suck on her breasts while making love. As mentioned earlier, a man can drink in his partner's yin energy from her lips and tongue, her breasts, and her vagina. The woman can also drink in her partner's yang energy from his lips, nipples, and penis. This energy exchange is balancing and healing for both partners.

In this position, a woman who has strengthened her PC muscle can stimulate the shaft of a man's penis and stimulate the reflexology points of his penis. By not stimulating the head of the penis, the couple can have sex for a very long time and can have extended orgasms. In chapter 2, we describe a number of exercises that a woman can use to stimulate herself and her partner with her PC muscle. A woman can squeeze and massage a man's penis with her PC muscle in any position, even when the man is on top.

In the woman-on-top position, she can direct the head of her partner's penis to the most sensitive parts of her vagina, including her G spot, which is one reason that for many women this is also the easiest position in which to have (multiple) orgasms.

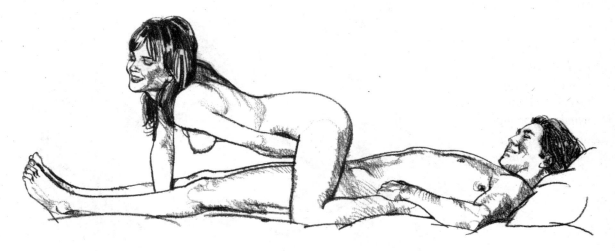

The woman can direct her partner's penis to her most sensitive spots and can use her PC muscle to stimulate his shaft.

Exercise 18

AROUND THE WORLD IN ONE NIGHT

1. During lovemaking, the woman straddles the man, facing him. She then squeezes her PC muscle around the shaft of the man's penis, without stimulating the head.

2. She moves up and down the shaft while he's inside her without pulling so far up that he comes out or that she squeezes around the head. She can move up and down on his penis for nine shallow thrusts and one deep thrust. This will be highly pleasurable for both.

3. She then does steps 1 and 2 again, only now with her back to him while facing his feet.

4. She then returns to facing him and squeezes up and down his penis. She can continue rotating as long as she likes.

MAN FROM BEHIND

In the man-from-behind position a woman's vagina is especially tight, and this position can be highly arousing both for men and for women. By squeezing her thighs together, the woman increases the tightness of her vagina and her ability to contract her PC muscle. In this position, and especially when the woman's torso is angled down or she lies flat (see illustration on p. 53), the woman's G spot is often easiest to reach. As a result, this position is extremely valuable for helping women experience multiple orgasms. When kneeling,

In this position a woman's vagina is especially tight, which can be highly arousing for both men and women.

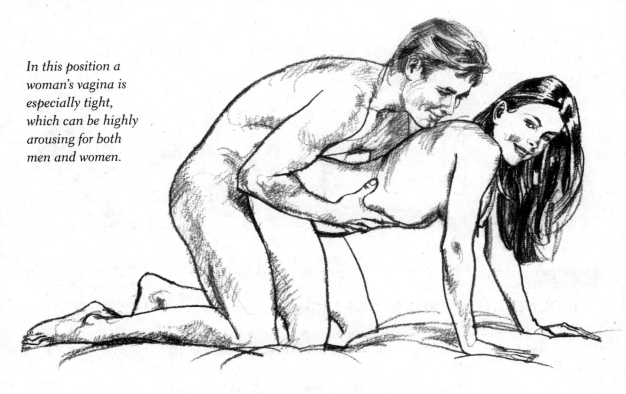

the man can also use a free hand to stimulate his partner's clitoris. When lying flat, the woman is probably better off stimulating her clitoris herself.

SIDE BY SIDE

The side-by-side position does not require much effort from either partner and is therefore good for later stages of lovemaking and for relaxing with each other after more vigorous lovemaking. The position is a little difficult to achieve and to maintain since penetration is generally shallow. It may be easiest to start with the man on top and to roll over into this position. Lying face-to-face with full-body contact is good for harmonizing and circulating energy.

SITTING POSITION

The sitting position is a variation of the woman-on-top position and a favorite for Healing Love. The parallel positioning and the close embrace make this an extremely intimate and healing position. This position is perfect for later lovemaking, soulful connection, and energy circulation.

If the woman leans back and supports herself on her arms, the couple can generate a great deal of friction in this position, but generally the position is best for less-vigorous thrusting. The thrusting, however, relies on the rocking of the pelvis, which can assist the circulation of energy up the spine. You can help your partner circulate the energy by stroking up his or her spine and drawing the energy down from the head to the abdomen.

The parallel positioning and the close embrace make the sitting position an extremely intimate and healing position.

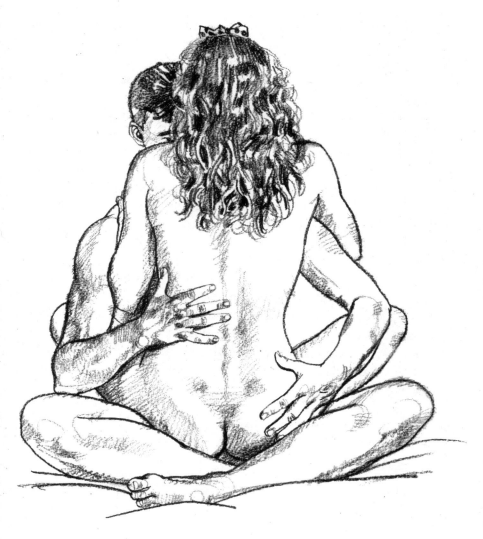

The sitting position is perfect for later lovemaking, soulful connection, and energy circulation.

STANDING POSITION

In a more strenuous but powerful adaptation of the previous position, the man stands while the woman wraps her legs around him (see illustration opposite). This position requires quite a bit of strength, coordination, and balance, but it can be extremely energizing. The ability to thrust in this position is limited (unless the woman is propped against a counter), but it is excellent for circulating and exchanging energy.

Circulating Sexual Energy

Circulating energy during lovemaking shifts the focus of intercourse from the often fun and frenetic race for orgasm to a more meditative process of making love.

As discussed in chapter 3, circulating sexual energy through your body is a powerful way to nourish your whole system and to transform the fleeting pleasure of orgasm into an enduring ecstatic experience that is profoundly healing. Circulating energy during lovemaking shifts the focus of intercourse from the often fun and frenetic race for orgasm to a more meditative process of making love.

In chapter 3, you learned how to circulate energy within your own body while alone. In this section, you will learn to circulate energy within your own body but now while making love with your partner. In chapter 7, you will learn how to give energy to your partner and to receive energy from your partner in the Soul-Mating exercise. This exchange of energy allows a profound level of healing and intimacy, but first we must understand how to circulate energy in our own body during lovemaking.

DRAWING UP AND GETTING DOWN

You can circulate sexual energy at any time from when you are first aroused to when you are close to orgasm. Circulating your energy will rejuvenate you and will help the man decrease his urge to ejaculate. Women and those men who have learned to separate orgasm from ejaculation can also circulate the energy during and after they orgasm. A man can still circulate energy after he ejaculates, but he will have much less energy to draw up, since he has poured much of his energy out through his ejaculation.

When you are both highly aroused, stop and hold each other. Look deeply into each other's eyes. Truly see your partner's inner goodness, and express the depth of your love with your eyes. Keeping your eyes open also helps bring the energy up.

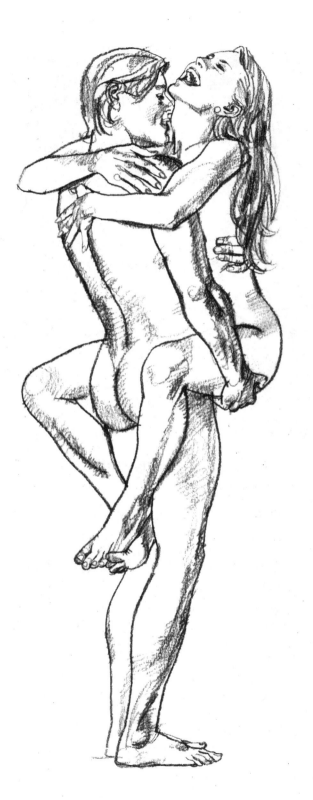

While thrusting is limited, the standing position is a powerful one for circulating energy.

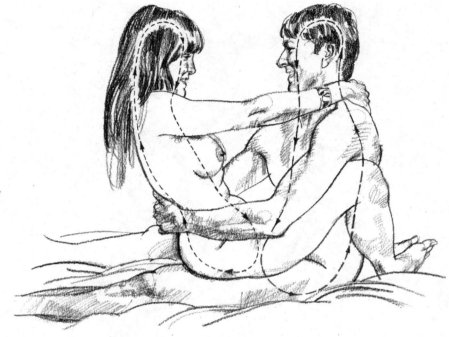

Couples must first learn to circulate sexual energy in their own body during lovemaking. Later, partners can learn to give and receive sexual energy.

Finding the Way

Three Levels of Cultivating Sexual Energy

- CIRCULATING BY YOURSELF: Circulate sexual energy within your own body while self-pleasuring.

- CIRCULATING IN YOUR OWN BODY WITH EACH OTHER: Circulate sexual energy within your own body while making love with your partner.

- CIRCULATING AND EXCHANGING WITH EACH OTHER: Exchange sexual energy with your partner while making love.

Exercise 19

THE ORGASMIC UPWARD DRAW DURING LOVEMAKING

1. STOP: When both of you are highly aroused, pull back so that the tip of the man's penis is just inside the entrance to the woman's vagina. This will allow both of you to cool down.

2. EXHALE AND CONTRACT: Each of you should exhale and contract your PC muscle. It may help for the man to contract first, so the force of the woman's PC muscle does not push him over the edge.

3. PUMP: Pump the energy back to the sacrum and up the spine to the crown of the head by contracting your PC muscle and anus.

4. REST AND SMILE: Rest and smile to the sexual organs, and let the energy rise up to your head.

5. SPIRAL: Spiral the energy in your head by rolling your eyes in circles nine times left and then right.

6. CIRCULATE: Bring the energy down the front of your body to your sexual organs with the Inner Smile. Continue circulating the energy up your spine and down your front.

7. MAKE LOVE: Continue to make love.

8. STORE: When you are done, touch your navel as you focus there. Smile and imagine the energy spiraling into your navel and being drawn down from your head to your abdomen, where it can be stored and released to nourish your body.

Relaxing during lovemaking also allows the hormone-filled blood from your genitals to return and fortify the rest of your body. Do not be concerned if the man's erection decreases. This is the only way that the blood can return to his body, and it will allow new blood to flow into his penis as he gets hard again once you continue making love.

Multi-Orgasmic Quickies and Marathons

For Taoists, the longer you make love, the more healing energy you are able to generate and circulate. The classic Taoist texts suggest that it takes a thousand loving thrusts to satisfy a woman completely. Before this starts to sound like a marathon, it is worth pointing out, as Jolan Chang does in his *Tao of Love and Sex*, that a half hour's jog takes at least two thousand steps. If

The classic Taoist texts suggest that it takes a thousand loving thrusts to satisfy a woman completely.

a half-hour jog should require two thousand steps, why should a half hour of lovemaking not involve a thousand loving thrusts?

This duration is quite different from that of most modern lovemaking. When Alfred Kinsey conducted his famous studies of human sexuality in the fifties, he found that average "coition" (that is, lovemaking) for an American couple was two minutes. The average has since risen to around ten minutes. The ancient Taoists would explain a great deal of the discontent in the modern bedroom with these figures. It is very difficult to fully satisfy and energize a couple—especially the woman—with such short lovemaking. While sex should not become a marathon or an endurance test, it is worth remembering that by Taoist standards our modern lovemaking is often far too brief to reach the heights—and depths—that can be experienced.

Of course, for most of us, our hectic life does not afford opportunities for prolonged lovemaking every night or even every week. Still, to reach the more profound and energizing levels of ecstatic lovemaking, we need to set aside time when we will not be interrupted by the phone, children, or anyone else. Staying home for an evening of lovemaking is certainly more entertaining than going out to the movies, and a weekend tryst can allow just the kind of break that our desire needs to be awakened fully.

Before you start worrying about how to fit hours of lovemaking into your life, it is worth mentioning multi-orgasmic quickies. When you and your partner start practicing Healing Love, you will find that your bodies are in tune and that you can experience heights of multi-orgasmic energetic lovemaking very quickly. Much will depend on how skillfully the female partner's sexual waters can be brought to a boil by her partner and herself, but, with the techniques described in the earlier chapters of this book, her desire can quickly be raised to a rapid boil.

Sex is many things, and while we strongly encourage you to explore the heights of Healing Love, we do not recommend that you abandon the more instinctual pleasures of heart-racing couplings. You may wish to think of Healing Love and especially the circulation of energy as a gourmet dinner that you anticipate and savor as often as your life affords but that you do not expect every night. When you choose a more feverish pace, you can still circulate your sexual energy once you are done and resting, although you will have less energy to draw up, especially the man if he has not yet learned to orgasm without ejaculating. Still, whenever you are having sex with love and a desire to heal each other, you are practicing Healing Love.

But when do we stop? Most people stop having sex when the man ejaculates and hopefully *after* the woman has had at least one orgasm. Once you

> When you and your partner start practicing Healing Love, you will find that your bodies are in tune and that you can experience heights of multi-orgasmic energetic lovemaking very quickly.

are both multi-orgasmic, there is no longer this obvious ending point. You and your partner will need to decide how long you want to make love and when you are satisfied. Most of us are not accustomed to paying close attention to our sexual appetites and knowing when we are really sexually satisfied. You and your partner will have to pay close attention to your desire and decide when you are both done.

The Taoists encouraged people to stop eating several bites before they are actually full. As the food descends to the stomach, a person will discover that he or she is pleasantly full and not uncomfortably stuffed. The Taoists similarly encouraged lovers to stop lovemaking before they are totally sated, to stop with their embers still burning. This remaining desire will allow you to continue to crave your partner the next night and the next night for a lifetime of passionate lovemaking.

Coming and Going

According to the Taoists, multiple orgasms are not the only reason a man should learn to orgasm without ejaculating. As we've mentioned, the Taoist masters were physicians and were therefore concerned with sexuality as part of the overall health of the body. Through their close observation, they discovered that ejaculation drains a man of his energy. Men usually notice this loss of energy in their own body as they long for sleep after ejaculating. Women are constantly lamenting their partner's disinterest in intimacy, conversation, or even cuddling after he ejaculates. The man who ejaculates, grunts, and falls asleep on top of his partner is regularly depicted in the media. The way that ejaculation exhausts a man's body was already well known several thousand years ago.

> After ejaculating, a man is tired, his ears buzz, his eyes are heavy, and he longs for sleep. He is thirsty and his limbs feel weak and stiff. In ejaculating he enjoys a brief moment of sensation but then suffers long hours of exhaustion.
>
> Peng-Tze, a sex adviser to the famed
> Yellow Emperor

Younger men will not feel the depletion as much as older men. And men who ejaculate after a long time will feel it much less than men who are ejaculating often. As we discussed in chapter 2, every time a man has an orgasm, he draws energy into his body. If he eventually ejaculates after having multiple

How depleted a man feels by ejaculation will depend on his age, his health, how often he ejaculates, and how energetic the lovemaking was before he ejaculated.

orgasms and especially after circulating energy, he will lose much less energy. How depleted a man feels by ejaculation will depend on his age, his health, how often he ejaculates, and how energetic the lovemaking was before he ejaculated.

If a man does not ejaculate, he will of course have much more energy to circulate. If he brings this energy down to his abdomen, the energy will be stored in his organs and released when his body needs it over the next twelve to fourteen hours. Many multi-orgasmic men and women who cultivate their energy describe feeling orgasms that last for hours after climax.

Many people who do not understand the difference between orgasm and ejaculation assume that the Taoist tradition warns men against having orgasms. We hope it is clear by now that men can have as many orgasms as they want as long as they learn to avoid ejaculating.

We discuss the effects of "going to seed" on a man's body at length in *The Multi-Orgasmic Man.* We encourage all men (and women) who want to know how and why ejaculation depletes a man's body to read it. The best proof, however, is in the man's own body. He can experiment easily in his own bedroom. See how much sleep he needs and how he feels the next morning after ejaculatory sex (especially after several nights of ejaculatory sex) and after non-ejaculatory, multi-orgasmic sex.

Unlike men, women generally do not have to worry about sex being depleting.

Unlike men, women generally do not have to worry about sex being depleting. The energy they lose through vaginal discharge during orgasm is minimal (even for those women who release a spray—often called female ejaculation—during intense orgasm). Of course, often after especially intense or "terminal" orgasms many women feel tired or "done." This feeling of completion comes from the release of orgasm (even an especially intense release) and is nothing to worry about. If a woman wants to avoid this feeling of tiredness or exhaustion, she can simply circulate her sexual energy up through her body.

According to the Tao, women lose far less energy through sex than they lose through menstruation and childbirth. The Taoists, therefore, developed practices to shorten the length of menstruation and to decrease the pain that many women experience during their periods. While these practices are beyond the scope of this book, they are discussed at length in Mantak and Maneewan Chia's book *Healing Love Through the Tao: Cultivating Female Sexual Energy.*

Strengthening Your Sex Organs

If couples want to have good sex, they need to have healthy sex organs. The healing lovemaking that we have described so far in this book will certainly energize your sex organs as well as the rest of your body. There is, however, a Taoist exercise that you can do to strengthen your prostate (if you are a man) and your uterus (if you are a woman).

While we tend to think of the penis and the vagina as our sex organs, much of our sexual energy and sexual ability comes for men from their prostate and for women from their uterus. You can try the following exercise if you want to cultivate these vital parts of your body. Doing this exercise will also generate a great deal of sexual energy that you can circulate through your body even when you are not making love or self-pleasuring.

Exercise 20

PROSTATE AND UTERUS STRENGTHENING

1. Sit at the edge of a chair or stand with your feet shoulder-width apart.

2. Exhale and suck your lower abdomen in.

3. As you exhale, gently push the fingers of one hand into your abdomen right above your pubic bone to feel the muscles flatten.

4. Suck up the lower abdominal muscle several times as if you were sucking through a straw although without inhaling through your mouth or nose. (As you suck up the abdominal muscles you will notice your anus and vulva or testicles will rise slightly. This sucking massages your prostate or uterus and creates a vacuum, which will draw more energy to your prostate or uterus. Don't be surprised if you make funny sounds as you suck up the lower abdomen. It is the result of the vacuum you have created and a sign that you are doing it correctly.)

5. Inhale into your abdomen. Your fingers will be pushed outward. The suction will draw the energy into your pelvis.

6. Exhale slowly through your teeth, hissing like a snake.

7. Keep your attention on your prostate or uterus as it warms up.

8. As you relax, the energy will rise up to your head. You can smile to your sex organs to assist the energy rising up through your spine to your brain.

9. Spiral the energy in your head nine times one way and then nine times in reverse.

10. Touch the tip of your tongue to the roof of your mouth just behind your top front teeth and let the energy descend down to your navel. You can imagine the energy spiraling into your navel to help you absorb it.

Safer Sex and Sexual Health

Even with the medical advances that have been made in treating AIDS recently, sexually transmitted diseases are here to stay. For this reason it is worth mentioning briefly the topic of safer sex. In addition, sexual health can dramatically affect the frequency and satisfaction of your lovemaking. It is difficult to focus on the heights of pleasure when you are worrying about or experiencing pain, so please take a moment to read this section.

Safer sex precautions are recommended for all new couples. Condoms should be used for intercourse or fellatio (see "The Art of Condoms"). Dental dams should be used for cunnilingus and latex gloves for vaginal or anal stimulation.

Simple office testing is available for HIV, hepatitis B and C, syphilis, gonorrhea, and chlamydia. Keep in mind that it may take up to six months after HIV infection for a person to test positive. You should use safer sex precautions for six months after a possible exposure and then be retested. If both tests are negative, there is little reason to worry as long as both partners are monogamous.

Certain STDs, such as herpes and the human papillomavirus (HPV), which is responsible for genital warts, can be transmitted by skin contact, with or without a condom. Both herpes and HPV are extremely common (occurring in 25 percent and 50 percent of the young adult population respectively). They are embarrassing but not usually dangerous and can be medically treated. Keep your lovemaking healing by being tested and taking safer sex precautions.

With non-ejaculatory sex there is less risk of exchanging bodily fluids. While this does not reduce the risk of contracting other sexually transmitted diseases such as herpes or HPV, it does reduce the risk of contracting HIV and hepatitis, which are transmitted through the exchange of bodily fluids. By not ejaculating, the man does not transfer as much bodily fluid to his partner. Also, by not ejaculating he does not draw in as much of her bodily fluid. A man's penis is a little like a turkey baster. When he ejaculates, he creates a low-pressure vacuum that can then draw in fluid from his partner. While non-ejaculatory sex decreases the exchange of bodily fluids, thereby making all sex safer, it is not truly "safer sex" unless you use a condom.

THE ART OF CONDOMS

1. THERE IS NO SUBSTITUTE: Always use a condom before vaginal or anal intercourse, unless you and your partner have been tested for sexually transmitted diseases (STDS) and are monogamous.

2. GOOD NEWS & BAD NEWS: The good news about condoms is that the decreased sensitivity that most men experience can help them control their urge to ejaculate. The bad news about condoms is that they do decrease sensitivity for most men. Some men actually have difficulty keeping an erection while wearing a condom. If this happens, the man or his partner should keep stroking his genitals while he puts on the condom. Putting a small amount of lubricant on his penis before putting on the condom will increase his sensitivity without causing the condom to slip off.

3. ORAL SEX: Always use a condom before the woman performs oral sex. In this case, your partner will probably want to use a "dry" condom, one that is not lubricated.

4. GETTING IT ON: Leave half an inch of space at the top of plain-tip condoms. Reservoir-tip condoms are designed to create this space. Make sure that the condom covers the entire penis and smooth the condom to squeeze out any air bubbles. If the man is uncircumcised, he should pull back his foreskin before putting on the condom.

5. LUBRICANT: Apply plenty of lubricant to the outside of the condom. (Not enough lubricant is one of the major reasons that condoms break.) Use only water-based lubricants; petroleum-based lubricants and oils can cause latex condoms, dams, or gloves to disintegrate.

6. AFTERWARD: After intercourse, withdraw while he is still erect and hold the base of the condom to make sure it does not slip off. Throw away the condom and, especially if the man has ejaculated, wash off his penis or put on a new condom before continuing to caress one another.

7. BREAKING: A condom generally slips off or breaks because it wasn't put on correctly, because sex was "too" vigorous, or because the condom was not held during withdrawal. If the condom breaks or comes off and the man has not ejaculated or if the tear is near the base of the condom, you probably don't need to worry. Just remove the broken condom and put on a new one. If the condom breaks after ejaculation, safe sex experts recommend that the woman urinate and insert spermicidal foam or jelly into her vagina to help destroy the sperm, viruses, and bacteria. She should leave the spermicide there for at least an hour. If you are concerned about pregnancy, the woman may wish to take the "morning after" pill, which she can obtain from a physician.

It is important to remember that even with non-ejaculatory sex, bodily fluids are still being exchanged (remember the pre-ejaculate that you were warned about in sex ed). This is also why non-ejaculatory sex is not a reliable form of birth control. Non-ejaculatory sex will simply make safe sex safer and will make whatever form of birth control you are using that much more effective. However, we want to stress that non-ejaculatory sex should not be relied on as a form of birth control alone.

The Power to Hurt and to Heal

HIV and other sexually transmitted diseases are a reminder of a powerful Taoist understanding: lovemaking is a physical and energetic exchange that can profoundly influence the health and well-being of both partners. The sexual revolution did not take into account this exchange, and we have yet to fully realize the extent to which we are influenced by our sexual history. The biochemical and energetic exchange that takes place through our sexual organs has profound physical, emotional, and even spiritual effects on both partners.

While the epidemic spread of AIDS and other sexually transmitted diseases may be new, the power of sex to heal and to hurt us is not. In our modern society, we tend to see sex in biological and relational terms: as a simple part of relationships between consenting adults. However, the Tao reminds us that sex is a sacred act with the power to bring illness and destruction or to bring healing and the creation of new life. The Tao sees lovemaking in characteristically pragmatic health terms, but it never loses its sense of respect and awe for this source of our life. In the next two chapters we will discuss how to keep lovemaking filled with intimacy and sacredness.

CHAPTER 6

Making Real Love

In this chapter you will discover:

- The Power of Sex to Intensify Our Emotions, Positively and Negatively

- How to Connect Love and Lust

- How to Cultivate Self-Love and Love for Each Other

- Touch Meditation

- How to Transform Negative Feelings Toward Your Partner with the Inner Smile

Healing Love not only allows greater sexual pleasure and health; it also leads to the potential for ever-deepening emotional intimacy. We call good sex "lovemaking," but really making "love" requires an understanding of the power of sexuality to heal—or wound—our heart.

We have said several times that sexual energy simply expands the energy in your body—positive or negative. We have tried to emphasize the need to feel love and to avoid anger. Let's look at this relationship between sexual energy and emotions more closely and explore what you can do to keep your Healing Love truly loving.

As you learn to practice Healing Love and to expand your sexual energy, it is essential that you cultivate loving-kindness toward yourself and your partner. The exercises in this chapter and the next will help you cultivate love and compassion. As you practice Healing Love, keep in mind that sexual energy is like fire. Fire can cook your food, or it can burn your house down. It all depends on how it is used. Sexual energy is the same.

It is essential that you transform your sexual energy into love and compassion or it can turn to anger and hate. The role of sexual energy in amplifying our emotions helps explain why lovers' quarrels are always the most explosive and why love and hate are so intimately connected. As you learn to generate more and more life-giving sexual energy, it is important that you connect it with the compassionate energy of your heart. Lust, for Taoists, is a vital part of our life-force energy, but it must be cultivated and connected to our love for our partner.

Cultivating Self-Love

The Taoists said and many psychologists today agree that we can't really love others until we can love ourselves. But what exactly does it mean to cultivate self-love, and why is it so important for a healthy sex life? First, it should be pointed out that self-love is quite different from egotism or narcissism. It is simply the feeling of love and acceptance of oneself. It is essential for a healthy sex life and love life because without self-love it is impossible to be a loving partner. Having compassion for oneself is essential for having compassion for our partner and for others in our life.

> **The Taoists knew that sexual energy simply expands the energy in your body—positive or negative.**

> **Sexual energy is like fire. Fire can cook your food, or it can burn your house down. It all depends on how it is used. Sexual energy is the same.**

> **Without self-love it is impossible to be a loving partner.**

Exercise 21

CONNECTING LOVE AND LUST

1. Touch your fingertips to your heart in the center of your chest.

2. Smile to your heart and feel it soften, and then imagine it blossoming like a red flower. Feel it fill with love, joy, and compassion for yourself.

3. Keep the fingertips of your left hand touching your heart, and place your right hand on your genitals.

4. Men should feel the energy moving from their genitals up to their heart and from their heart back to their genitals. Women should feel the energy moving from their heart down to their genitals and then back to their heart. (In addition to connecting love and lust, the heart energy, which is like fire, will heat the yin "waters" of her vagina and help her become aroused.)

5. Imagine the times of most intimate lovemaking with your partner or when you are feeling most loving toward your partner. This will allow you to gain access to this Healing Love and to combine your love and lust.

The intimacy of sex can bring up our greatest insecurities about ourselves. Many of us worry about our body and about our attractiveness to our partner. Our body is not perfect, but we assume it should be. Beyond our own lover, we rarely see other bodies that are not airbrushed by the advertising industry. We hold ourselves up to standards that are truly unrealistic and unhelpful to our own self-acceptance. Those who regularly see different people naked, like physicians or massage therapists, know that there are really no perfect bodies and that every body has its own beauty.

Sex also brings up our insecurities about our skills in bed. Since none of us are schooled in the Arts of the Bedchamber, we remain very insecure about our knowledge and our skills. Admitting to ourselves and to our partner that we are all just learning what pleases us and what pleases our partner is the first step to transcending this insecurity. Fear, anxiety, and nervousness are three of the bedfellows most able to sabotage our sex life. A sense of playfulness and even laughter can help to break the bedroom worries and allow us to see that our lover is our playmate and loving companion on the path to sexual satisfaction.

The following exercise will help you to connect with your partner and to convey your appreciation and love for her or his unique body. It is a very powerful exercise when one of you is feeling insecure, when you have been apart, or when you are trying to rebuild trust in your relationship.

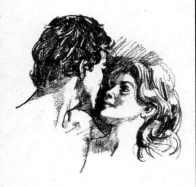

Looking into each other's eyes is a powerful way to connect and to send Healing Love.

Exercise 22

NINE FLOWERS TOUCH MEDITATION

1. LOOK INTO EACH OTHER'S EYES: Sit comfortably facing each other and looking into each other's eyes.

2. TOUCH YOURSELF: Decide who will go first. If you go first, you should use both hands to touch your own body, generally from head to toe. (Avoid any parts of your body that you do not want your partner to touch, and generally leave your genitals for last.) As you touch each part of your body, feel compassion and acceptance for it.

3. YOUR PARTNER FOLLOWS: Your partner should use his or her hands to follow, lovingly touching each place that you have just touched.

4. SMILE AND SEND LOVE: When you are finished, your partner should smile and send you love and acceptance with his or her eyes. If you wish, the one who has followed can convey his or her love verbally, such as, "This is the body of my beloved," or "I love every inch of this body." Focus your comments on your love for your partner and not just on your lust.

5. SWITCH: Then switch roles.

6. EXPLORE YOURSELF: Now together lightly touch your own nipple very gently, using a featherlight touch. Barely touch it. Now spiral from the nipple out around the nipple and circling about a half inch away from the nipple (at the edge of the dark skin or areola). Circle around the nipple eighteen, thirty-six, or more times. You will feel an itchy, aroused feeling as your sexual energy expands.

7. MAKE NINE CIRCLES: Now move down about one-half to one inch and make another circle, as if you are drawing a flower. Continue moving down the body from the nipple to the genitals, making circles about one-half to one inch apart. You are exploring your body and connecting the breast or heart to the genitals. The ninth circle should be at your pubis right above your sexual organs.

8. EXPLORE EACH OTHER: The man should then make nine circles on the woman, and then the woman should do it back to the man.

9. MAKE HEALING LOVE: Now make love however you and your partner wish with your whole bodies and your whole hearts.

This touch meditation requires slowness and patience, which can often be difficult for a man's rapid sexual response, or, as the Taoists put it, "yang fire." Men need to learn how to contain their fire and to keep it burning low. As they are able to control their fire, they will avoid burning out their sexual energy too quickly and ejaculating. The man should relax, smile, and draw the energy up. He should focus on igniting the woman's passion into a roiling boil. Once the woman's desire is boiling, the man's fire will ignite quickly and both partners will be ready for lovemaking.

Cultivating Love for Each Other

How to cultivate love in a relationship is a profound subject, and we could not possibly summarize it in a few paragraphs. In addition, this is a book about sex more than love, although the Taoists have always known that for profound and healing sex, you can never separate the two.

Emotions like anger and irritation inevitably limit our affection and attraction for our partner. The Taoists recognized that anger and irritation can create disharmony in the bedroom and in the relationship. They also believed that anger and other negative emotions were toxic to our bodies and health. They strongly recommended avoiding the lovers' quarrels and fiery confrontations that characterize many modern relationships. Instead, they recommended the path of gentleness and compassion.

The Tao values humility and flexibility and symbolizes these qualities in water, which always seeks the lowest place and always changes to fit its container. The Taoists also admired the patience and power of water. They noticed that a river, while humble and flexible enough to move around great boulders, would inevitably wear these boulders away in time.

Every relationship will experience the inevitable stresses and strains of partnered life, and each couple will choose their own way to address them. There is a simple exercise that echoes the Taoist qualities of gentleness and compassion and that emulates the complementary relationship of yin and yang. Many couples have used it to help them understand and harmonize with each other.

Each partner takes a turn listening to what is upsetting his or her partner and then repeats what was said. This refocuses us away from our hurt and toward understanding the pain of our partner. It also allows us to know that our partner has heard what is painful for us.

Exercise 23

LISTENING WITH LOVE

1. HOLD HANDS: Begin by holding hands.

2. LISTEN WITH COMPASSION: Your partner takes a few minutes to explain what is upsetting him or her while you listen quietly. As you listen, smile and let your heart soften and fill with compassion. Try to send loving energy to your partner.

3. REPEAT WHAT YOU HEARD: When your partner is done, you then repeat what you heard. Obviously, you do not need to repeat every word, just the main points. If you did not hear it all, repeat what you heard and invite your partner to tell you again whatever you have missed.

4. EXPRESS YOUR OWN FEELINGS: Then it is your turn to express what is upsetting you. Avoid engaging in an argument or attacking your partner. Simply describe what has been hurtful. It is important to express your hurt without getting defensive and without attacking. Talk about how you feel rather than what your partner has done. The more vulnerable you can be with each other, the more your hearts will open and the more compassionate you will be.

Staying in Touch

Fortunately, our biology can also help us during difficult times. In chapter 4, "Pleasuring Each Other," we discussed the power of touch to bond and arouse us during times of loving intimacy. Touch is equally important during the difficult times that occur in all relationships. The hormones that are released during touch can have a profound effect on our feelings toward our partner. As Theresa Crenshaw points out, "Withholding touch at a crucial moment can break a relationship. Maintaining continuity of touch during troubled times can save one."[1]

Touch literally keeps us "in touch" and can decrease our frustrations with and anger toward the other. For this reason, holding hands, which increases oxytocin, can help when discussing difficult topics. This is also part of the value of the Nine Flowers Touch Meditation when you are feeling a need to reconnect with each other's bodies.

Love Lies Within

Using our hormones can keep us bonded, but love is much more than chemistry. Still, according to the Tao, the secret to love also lies within. People frequently say they are "looking" for love or they have "fallen" in love, as if love were dependent on their partner apart from themselves. We too often look outside ourselves for love rather than nurturing our own source of loving energy. For Taoists, however, love is a physical energy of the heart, not just a mental emotion. They therefore tried to cultivate love within themselves quite independent of their partner.

Cultivating love is a noble goal, but what do we do with all of our negative emotions, like anger and resentment, which are bound to arise in any intimate relationship? Most of us dump our emotions on our partner and others, like we dump our garbage. We scream, we blame, we accuse, we belittle, we withdraw, and then we make up or we break up. It is easy to find fault with our partner or to conclude that something is wrong with the relationship.

With most relationships, Taoists believed, our love for our partner is less dependent on our partner and on the relationship than it is on our own capacity for love. According to the Tao, there is an alternative to either suppressing our emotions or venting them on our partner. We can cultivate them. Instead of dumping our emotional garbage, we recycle it.

The Taoists taught many psychospiritual exercises for recycling negative emotions, but in chapter 3 you learned one of the simplest and most effective: the Inner Smile. Today, Western medicine has shown through many studies that stress has negative effects on the immune system and has confirmed the debilitating effects of so-called toxic emotions, like anger. The Inner Smile is an easy way to cultivate and recycle these toxic emotions.

You can do the Inner Smile discussed in chapter 3 and also recycle your negative emotions through the following exercise. Just as we associate love with the heart (the reason for all those heart-shaped cards on Valentine's Day), the Taoists associated each emotion with one of our organs. For Taoists, as we mentioned above, our emotions are more than mere mental constructs. They are physical energies that are centered in particular organs, and we can most effectively work with these emotions by working with the energy of these organs.

For the Taoists, love is a physical energy of the heart, not just a mental emotion. They therefore tried to cultivate love within themselves quite independent of their partner.

Finding the Way

Emotional Chart

POSITIVE EMOTIONS	NEGATIVE EMOTIONS	ORGAN
Love, Joy, Compassion	Hatred, Impatience	Heart
Openness, Acceptance	Worry	Spleen
Courage	Sadness, Depression	Lungs
Gentleness, Calmness	Fear	Kidneys
Kindness, Generosity	Anger, Frustration	Liver

If you have a frequent problem with a particular negative emotion like anger, sadness, hate, fear, impatience, arrogance, or worry, you may wish to try the Six Healing Sounds, which help to cultivate and transform particular emotions. An extended discussion of the Inner Smile and the Six Healing Sounds can be found in Mantak Chia's *Taoist Ways to Transform Stress into Vitality*.

For Taoists, our emotions are physical energies centered in particular organs.

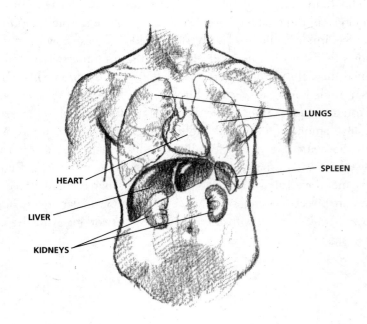

| Exercise 24 |

RECYCLING OUR NEGATIVE EMOTIONS

1. Touch your fingertips to your heart in the center of your chest.

2. Smile to your heart (smiling with both your mouth and your eyes), and feel it blossoming like a red flower. Feel it fill with love, joy, and compassion for yourself. (If you have difficulty feeling these emotions for yourself, envision a child, parent, grandparent, or friend for whom you feel love, joy, and compassion.)

3. Touch your spleen on your left-hand side under your rib cage, and smile to the spleen and feel openness and acceptance replace worry.

4. Touch your lungs, and feel courage replace sadness and depression.

5. Touch your kidneys (on your back opposite your navel on both sides of the spine), and feel gentleness, calmness, and stillness replace fear and nervousness.

6. Touch the liver on the right-hand side under the rib cage, and feel kindness and generosity replace anger and frustration.

7. Now see your partner's face, and smile and send loving energy to your partner.

Power and Compassion

The Healing Love practices that expand your sexual energy are very powerful. As they expand their sexual energy and learn greater skill in bed, it is quite common for people to develop greater self-confidence in bed. Men especially need to be careful not to let this greater prowess go to their head. Power is about conquest and is the opposite of love. As with any martial art, the real secret of power in Sexual Kung Fu is not ego or hardness but egolessness and softness. To practice Healing Love, both men and women need to open their hearts and practice with a spirit of love and humility. Only with this openness of your body and your heart can you truly feel the flow of energy within you and between you and your partner.

PLAYING BY HEART

Remember not to put your practice before your partnership. If any of the Healing Love practices make you feel awkward in bed, you can practice them by yourself until they become natural. Men especially need time to learn how to separate orgasm from ejaculation and how to use their breath and

Without your sincere love for each other, sex is simply friction. Friction is certainly pleasurable, but it is real love that will bind your bodies together in ecstatic lovemaking for a lifetime.

their PC muscle. Make sure you stay present with your partner. The techniques that you learn in this book are simply that—techniques. You need to learn the techniques well enough so that you can forget them. Just as with learning to play a musical instrument, you will first need to learn each of the notes, but eventually you will be able to play from the heart. Learning to make love from the heart is the essence of Healing Love. Without your sincere love for each other, sex is simply friction. Friction is certainly pleasurable, but it is real love that will bind your bodies together in ecstatic lovemaking for a lifetime.

In the next chapter, we will discuss how the compassion that you cultivate during Healing Love can deepen your spiritual relationship and your spiritual life as a whole.

CHAPTER 7

Sexing the Spirit

In this chapter you will discover:

- The Importance of Your Sexuality for Your Spiritual Growth and Spiritual Life

- Energizing Morning Prayer Lovemaking

- Soul-Mating and Soul Orgasms

- How to Make Your Sexual Energy Most Powerful and Nourishing

- How to Transform Sexual Energy into Spiritual Energy

- Cultivating the Highest Form of Life Energy

- The Profound Connection Between Your Relationship and the World

Sexuality and spirituality are inextricably linked for Taoists.

Sexuality and spirituality are inextricably linked for Taoists. For this reason sexuality is seen as an essential part of the spiritual path. In the West, we have torn ourselves in two: a fleshy, sinful body and an immaterial, saintly soul. For the Taoists this separation is artificial. Indeed, Taoist sexuality allows us to experience an embodied, palpable spirituality. The soul itself is said to reside at the navel in the abdomen, and it is believed that high levels of orgasmic energy allow the soul to emerge. You probably didn't hear *that* in Sunday school.

For Taoists, sexual energy is sacred. Whenever we are aroused, whenever we are having sex, we are in communion with the divine, or universal, energy. But most people do not know how to use this energy to cultivate their spiritual life.

Sadly, most of the world's religious systems regard sex as negative or even evil and therefore try to suppress it. Even when they do not suppress it, religious traditions generally consider sex as a distraction or a hindrance along the spiritual path. Most people have been taught that they have to deny their sexuality to grow spiritually. According to the Tao, this is misguided. Sexual energy makes up approximately a quarter of our total life force. People who deny sexual energy lose access to this vital source of energy and vitality for their life *and* their spiritual growth.

Sexual energy makes up approximately a quarter of our total life force. People who deny sexual energy lose access to this vital source of energy and vitality for their life *and* their spiritual growth.

Morning Prayer

The Taoists developed a simple way to cultivate this vital life energy each morning, and they saw it as so essential to their spiritual as well as their physical well-being that they called it "Morning Prayer."

We tend to think of sex as a nighttime activity and relegate our love life to the moments before we go to bed. The Taoists knew this is often not an ideal time for lovemaking because we are often exhausted from the day and our bodies long for sleep as much as for sex. While Healing Love at night before bed can be very energizing and allow us to sleep more soundly and wake more refreshed, the Taoists thought that morning lovemaking is equally if not more important for starting the day off right.

Even brief lovemaking in the morning was considered to be extremely energizing because it allows us to greet the day and its inevitable frustrations with a lighthearted and joyous spirit. Try it, and you will find that it is better than caffeine. But remember, it is essential that the man avoid ejaculating, or he will lose much of his energy.

Exercise 25

MORNING PRAYER

1. Make love however you find arousing and satisfying.

2. As you approach orgasm or after you have had one or more orgasms, circulate the energy throughout your body with the Orgasmic Upward Draw.

3. Circulate the energy down to your navel with the Inner Smile.

4. Continue lovemaking and circulating the energy until you are sexually satisfied and physically energized.

When you are not able to practice Morning Prayer, you can always begin your day by circulating your own energy through the Inner Smile and the Orgasmic Upward Draw. Eventually you will be able to feel an energizing, even orgasmic, wave of energy anytime and anywhere. Now *that* could really improve your commute. Once you have learned to circulate energy in your own body, you are ready for soul-mating.

Union: Soul-Mating and Soul Orgasms

In Exercise 19: The Orgasmic Upward Draw During Lovemaking, in chapter 5, you learned to circulate energy in your own body during lovemaking. In Soul-Mating you actually exchange energy with your partner. This experience is profoundly intimate and can lead to a feeling of union and oneness that is difficult to describe and profound to experience.

When both partners experience the intense energy exchange of Soul-Mating, they are able to feel orgasmic pleasure for many hours and to feel deeply connected to their partner even when they are apart. This is what the Taoists call a Soul Orgasm.

Because Healing Love teaches couples to circulate energy to each other beyond simple physical touch, they are able to feel this electrical connection even when they are not touching or are not together. When both partners are feeling highly orgasmic, their souls begin to emerge and can join together above their heads. Once joined beyond their physical bodies, they are able to maintain this union long after lovemaking.

Couples are able to feel orgasmic pleasure for many hours and to feel deeply connected to their partners even when they are apart.

Helpful Hints for Soul-Mating

- FACE-TO-FACE: For this exercise, as in the Orgasmic Upward Draw During Lovemaking, it is best to be in a face-to-face position with most of your bodies in contact. If the woman is much lighter she should be on top; otherwise, it doesn't matter which partner is on top. The sitting position is one of the best for exchanging sexual energy.

- SEND HEALING LOVE WITH YOUR EYES: It is very helpful when you are exchanging energy to look into each other's eyes. Through your eyes, you can send each other healing and loving energy. Remember to keep your genitals connected and hearts open at all times.

- TOUCHING TONGUES TO CLOSE THE CIRCUIT: When you touch tongues, you will be closing the circuit between your bodies.

- DRAWING YOUR SOULS OUT: You want to make sure that you have enough sexual energy to circulate and exchange. Wait until both of you are highly aroused but before the man is on the verge of ejaculating. If either or both of you are multi-orgasmic, you can enjoy several orgasms before soul-mating.

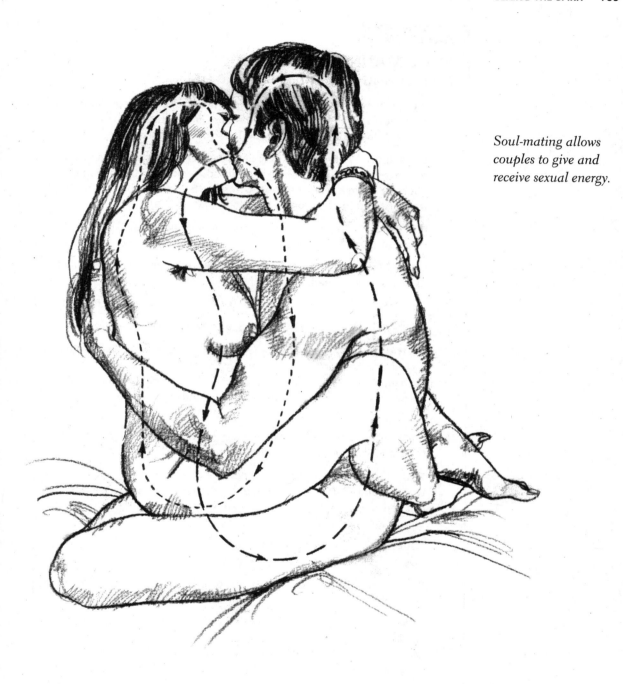

Soul-mating allows couples to give and receive sexual energy.

SOUL-MATING
EXCHANGING SEXUAL ENERGY AND HAVING SOUL ORGASMS

1. STOP: When the two of you are highly aroused, draw back slightly so that the tip of the man's penis remains inside the entrance to the woman's vagina. This will allow both partners to cool down.

2. EXHALE AND THEN CONTRACT: Each partner should exhale and then contract your PC muscle. Make sure that the woman's contraction does not push the man over the edge. Often it is helpful for the man to contract first and for the woman to follow.

3. PUMP: Pump the energy back to the sacrum and up the spine to the crown of the head by contracting your PC muscle and anus.

4. SMILE: Rest and smile to the sexual organ, and let the energy continue rising up to your head.

5. SPIRAL: Spiral the energy in your head by rolling your eyes from side to side.

6. THRUST: Continue to make love, stopping to circulate the energy.

7. EXCHANGE: When you are ready to exchange energy, the woman should send her partner cool yin energy from her vagina and absorb hot yang energy from his penis. At the same time, the man should send his partner his hot yang energy from his penis and absorb his partner's cool yin energy from her vagina.

8. CIRCULATE: Draw your partner's energy back to your spine and up to the crown of your head (contracting your PC muscle if necessary).

9. TOUCH TONGUES: Let the energy descend down the front of your head to your tongue. Touch your tongues together, which will close the circuit and allow the energy to be exchanged through your mouths as well as through your genitals.

10. LOVE: Bring the energy down to your heart, and exchange the healing love energy directly through your chests.

11. STORE: Smile as you focus on your navel and bring the energy down to your abdomen.

12. JOIN: Instead of leaving it in your navel as you did in the Orgasmic Upward Draw, you will keep the energy circulating around your Microcosmic Orbit and exchange it with your partner three, six, or nine times. Finally, imagine this refined, orgasmic, sexual-spiritual energy joining above your head with the energy of your partner. You can picture the image of your partner and you in sexual union above your head. This will allow your soul to unite with your partner's.

Universal Love

The Healing Love practice allows people to circulate their sexual energy and learn to multiply and expand their orgasms and their energy. In the previous chapters, you have learned how pleasurable, how healing, and how emotionally intimate this can be. You have learned how to generate sexual energy and how to transform it into physically and emotionally healing energy.

You may never have thought (or been taught) that so much joy and such profound power lay waiting in your sexual organs. Still, for the Taoists there was more. This sexual energy that you have learned to cultivate can be transformed into spiritual energy that allows you to transform yourself and your relationship—not only with your partner but also with the world.

The passion and compassion that you develop with your partner through Healing Love can profoundly affect your relationship to your partner and to others in your life. According to the Taoists, this love and ecstasy that we feel in our most intimate relationship is simply a taste of the Universal Love and the blissful oneness with the Original Force of the Universe that we can experience as we grow spiritually.

Unlike many spiritual traditions, the Tao does not valorize the spiritual benefits of Healing Love over the sexual, healing, or emotional benefits. Indeed, they are all simultaneous and complementary. We have organized the book with the spiritual practice at the end because in our bodies there is a continuum of energy from the most palpable, which is sexual energy (*ching chi*), to the most subtle, which is spiritual energy (*shen*).

There is also a natural progression from our sexual life to our emotional life to our spiritual life. If we are not able to cultivate our sexual life or our emotional life before we embark on a spiritual path, we will find that our spiritual progress is often undermined by our suppressed sexual desires and emotional needs. This is the unfortunate reason that so many spiritual leaders are found to have secret sexual lives that they have forbidden for their followers. They have not yet learned to integrate their sexual and emotional lives. The Tao sees that all of us are human, even our leaders, and that we cannot escape from the fact that we are embodied creatures with physical as well as spiritual needs.

If we are not able to cultivate our sexual life or our emotional life before we embark on a spiritual path, we will find that our spiritual progress is often undermined by our suppressed sexual desires and emotional needs.

Transforming Sexual Energy into Spiritual Energy

Sexual energy can be turned into spiritual energy by circulating the energy through your body along the Microcosmic Orbit that you learned about in chapter 3 and that you used to cultivate your sexual energy in prior chapters. Taoists said that circulating sexual energy through the body nine times (their sacred number) transforms it into spiritual energy. In addition, this refines the energy and makes it easier for your body to store and assimilate.

When sexual energy and loving energy are combined, the energy becomes stable and nourishing.

Equally important to creating spiritual energy is love. Remember, for Taoists, love is much more than an ephemeral feeling or mental construct. It is a bodily energy that is centered at the heart. When sexual energy (from your genitals) and loving and compassionate energy (from your heart) are combined, the energy becomes stable and nourishing. This energy will allow you, your relationship to your partner, and your relationship to the world to deepen and grow spiritually.

Compassion and the Virtues of Our Spiritual Life

The quality of our energy (chi) is just as important as the quantity. While the practices in this book will allow you to expand the energy in your life manifold, it is essential that this energy be positive rather than negative. The way to expand our positive energy is through cultivating our emotional and spiritual qualities, or what the Taoists called the Virtues. We discussed this briefly in the last chapter, on cultivating the positive emotions in our romantic relationship. In this section, we will expand on this discussion and explain the importance of cultivating these positive qualities in our life and relationships overall.

The Taoists believed that we are all born with the virtues of love, gentleness, kindness, respect, honesty, fairness, justice, and righteousness. These are actually the positive qualities of our emotions, and, characteristically for the embodied perspective of the Taoists, these qualities are all connected with the bodily organs. When we are expressing these virtues our life force energy (chi) flows smoothly and efficiently. If we neglect to cultivate these virtues, however, we run the risk of channeling our additional sexual energy directly into our negative emotions, exacerbating any negative or neurotic tendency we may have. (Keep in mind that we usually exude the emotional energies that are most prevalent within us.)

While we are born virtuous, emotions such as fear, anger, cruelty, impatience, worry, sadness, and grief are inevitable as we grow up. These emotions, if left to fester, can damage our health and weaken our immune system. Modern medicine now acknowledges that the presence of negative emotions like anger and fear can wear down the body's immune system before any clinical evidence of disease appears. These emotions can also pollute our individual relationships and our overall relationship with the world.

Some spiritual traditions urge us to get rid of these negative emotions and negative energy. Just as the Taoist practice does not suppress sexuality and sexual energy, it does not try to suppress these negative emotions and this negative energy. Negative emotions are a natural and inevitable part of being human, like day and night, hot and cold, or black and white. We can no more escape this emotional garbage than we can escape creating actual garbage. For Taoists, it is all energy. Their solution was to recycle these negative emotions and this negative energy into positive emotions and positive or virtuous energy. There is valuable energy in our negative emotions, just as there is great energy in our recycled garbage. For Taoists, nothing is wasted.

In the last chapter, you learned how to recycle and cultivate your negative emotions and negative energy into positive emotions and positive energy. By transforming hate into love, sadness and depression into courage, worry into openness, fear into gentleness, and anger into kindness, we literally detoxify our body, our emotions, and our spirit.

> **By transforming hate into love, sadness and depression into courage, worry into openness, fear into gentleness, and anger into kindness, we literally detoxify our body, our emotions, and our spirit.**

Cultivating Compassion

For the Taoists, compassion is the highest expression of human emotion and virtuous energy. Compassion is not a single virtue but the culmination of all virtues, expressed at any given moment as a blend of fairness, kindness, gentleness, honesty, respect, courage, and love. When a person is compassionate he or she has the power to express any or all of these virtues at the appropriate moment.

It should be pointed out that compassion is often misunderstood to be based on sympathy. According to the Tao, sympathy is a weakness individuals show when they are easily affected by the emotions of others. Compassion is more closely related to empathy, which is a superior state that can acknowledge the emotional outpourings of others without being thrown off balance by them. The difference between empathy and compassion, however, is that compassion is not seen as an emotion or a feeling but as a higher state of consciousness that naturally radiates the best human qualities. In short, the Taoists regarded compassion as the finest form of life energy.

Before we can truly open our heart and the rest of ourselves to our partner and to others in our life, we must make sure that we transform the negative emotions that we carry and cultivate compassion for ourselves, our partner, and others in our life. As you cultivate self-love and love for your partner, you can also take this love into the rest of your life. With compassion, one can love unconditionally and thereby accept the world on its own terms without suffering.

As you do "The Compassion Cycle" exercise below, remember to relax and breathe. Relaxing and breathing deeply will allow your body to open and make it easier for you to circulate and join the energies in your body. (For the location of your organs, see illustration on p. 162.)

> With compassion, one can love unconditionally and thereby accept the world on its own terms without suffering.

Exercise 27

THE COMPASSION CYCLE

1. YOUR HEART: Start by focusing on your heart. Smile to your heart, and let it feel soft and loving. With your mind, spiral this energy of love in your heart.

2. YOUR KIDNEYS: Now move your awareness to your kidneys (on your back opposite your navel on both sides of the spine). Smile to them, and let a feeling of gentleness rise up to your heart. Spiral this energy in your heart so that it blends with the energy of love already there.

3. YOUR LIVER: Now move your awareness to your liver (on your right-hand side under your rib cage). Smile to it, and let the feeling of kindness rise up to your heart. Spiral this energy in your heart so that it blends with the rest of the energy there.

4. YOUR HEART AGAIN: Now become aware of your heart again. Smile to it, and this time feel love, joy, and happiness. Spiral this energy in your heart so that it blends with the rest of the energy there.

5. YOUR SPLEEN: Now move your awareness to your spleen (on your left-hand side under your rib cage). Smile to it and let the feeling of openness and fairness rise up to your heart. Spiral this energy in your heart so that it blends with the rest of the energy.

6. YOUR LUNGS: Finally, move your awareness to your lungs. Smile to them, and let the feelings of courage and righteousness flow to your heart. Spiral this energy in your heart so that it blends with the rest of the energy and together becomes compassion energy.

Revealing Ourselves

For the Taoists, the microcosm (our body, our relationship) is inextricably linked to the macrocosm (the planet, the rest of humanity). As we heal and transform ourselves and our most intimate relationship, we heal and transform all our relationships and the world as a whole.

In *The Multi-Orgasmic Man*, we explained that the more pleasure we give, the more pleasure we receive. The more we heal, the more we are healed. In *The Multi-Orgasmic Couple*, we have tried to show that the more we open ourselves up physically, emotionally, and spiritually to our partner, the more pleasurable and profound our lovemaking and our relationship will be. The more we reveal ourselves, the more joy and love we can share with each other and with the world.

Multiple orgasms are part of an unfolding process of "becoming one" with each other and with the world. According to the Tao and even according to modern physics, the world is continually pulsating. When we orgasm, we harmonize not only with our partner but also with the world and its pulsations. It is for this reason that sexuality is seen as so vital to our physical, emotional, *and* spiritual health. The more we open ourselves and become one with our partner, the more we open ourselves and become one with the world. In the next chapter, we will discuss how to maintain this pleasure and love, this joy and harmony, for a lifetime in our most intimate relationship.

The more we open ourselves up physically, emotionally, and spiritually to our partner, the more pleasurable and profound our lovemaking and our relationship will be. The more we reveal ourselves, the more joy and love we can share with each other and with the world.

CHAPTER 8

Making Love for a Lifetime

In this chapter you will discover:

- Ways to Harmonize Differences in Your Desire

- Strategies for Waxing and Waning Desire

- Sexual Health for Older Women, Older Men, and Older Couples

- The Soft Entry Technique to Overcome Erection Problems

- How to Maintain the Sexual Charge in Your Relationship

- The Real Secret of Sexuality

In the West, we tend to think that passion peaks on the wedding night. Afterward, according to this cultural assumption, passion and sexual pleasure slowly decrease over the years until we accept our sexual dissatisfaction or seek other partners. This, the Taoists knew, does not have to be the case. In fact, for them the wedding night is just the beginning of a lifetime of ever more pleasurable and satisfying lovemaking as we learn the subtleties of our partner's body, emotions, mind, and spirit. Multiple orgasms, in particular, become easier for men and for many women as they get older. Experiencing the heights of Healing Love also becomes easier as you and your partner grow together physically, emotionally, and spiritually.

This chapter discusses the cycles that all couples experience as their desire for each other and what they need from each other change over months and years. Taoist sexuality is not about the thrill of the new but the thrill of the known. The Taoists understood that the potential for knowing one's partner is infinite since we, like the universe itself, are constantly changing.

Taoist sexuality is not about the thrill of the new but the thrill of the known. The Taoists understood that the potential for knowing one's partner is infinite since we, like the universe itself, are constantly changing.

The Waxing and Waning of Desire

While it is natural for each of us to continually change and grow over the course of our lifetime, these changes can be surprising and even frightening to us and to our partner. In particular, as our desire waxes and wanes with the cycles of family, work, and health, it is important to learn how to accommodate our sexual relationship without feelings of mistrust or betrayal.

For most of us our sexual relationship is the place where we are most vulnerable. It is difficult not to personalize our partner's sexual response. Men and women often take their partner's waning interest in sex as a judgment or criticism. It is important to remember that this is generally a cycle and not a cliff. Both men's and women's sex drives are dependent on hormones, which are constantly ebbing and flowing in our bodies. Family and health issues can also dampen one's sex drive for periods of time. With this said, it is important to discuss these sexual fluctuations and to avoid letting them go on for long periods of time without exploring their source.

This is important for both emotional and physiological reasons. Emotionally, it is important to avoid the lasting hurt and mistrust that can come from a partner's cold shoulder. Hormonally, as we discussed in chapter 4, the more sex your body has, the more sex your body wants. The longer we go without sexual contact, the easier it is to lose contact with our sexual self. Finally, it is important physiologically to keep the pipes working, especially as we get older.

The difficulty, of course, is what to do when one of you is feeling frisky and the other is frowning. Here is a list of options that can save your sex life and even the love and trust in the relationship. The Taoists have always known that when there is disharmony in the bedroom, there can never be harmony in the relationship. So resolving these times of disharmony and conjugal conflicts is essential for the well-being and happiness of your relationship as a whole.

Harmonizing Different Desires

What do you do when one of you is feeling sexual and the other is not?

It is essential to establish open and honest communication about the cycles of desire each of you experience. Often it is possible for this communication to rely on body language, but it is very easy to misunderstand or not fully to understand our partner's body. Rather than turning over with disappointment and hurt, it is essential to convey verbally our desire and to invite our partner to convey his or her desire.

There are various satisfying options for exchanging sexual energy even when one of you is not interested in intercourse or even being "sexual." It is important to remember that Healing Love is much more than multiple orgasms. There are several ways that can help ensure the quality of your sexual and overall relationship.

1. If you initiate sex, you must not take the highs and lows of your partner's sexual energy personally or as a reflection of your own attractiveness or desirability. This is very difficult to do. From our earliest experiences with romance and relationship on the adolescent dance floor, we take others' interest as a sign of our attractiveness and desirability as a partner. As we discussed in chapter 6, "Making Real Love," the Taoists knew that love has more to do with our own ability to love than it does with how lovable our partner is. Similarly, attraction has more to do with our own level of sexual energy than it does with how attractive our partner is. In other words, to feel desire or attraction to anyone, we must have access to our own sexual energy.

Attraction has more to do with our own level of sexual energy than it does with how attractive our partner is.

In our more external culture, where we are constantly barraged by images of airbrushed beauty, of silicone-enhanced breasts and washboard stomachs, it is hard not to feel that if we or our partner were more attractive, we or they would have more desire. Contrary to popular opinion, sexual energy is first and foremost generated in an individual's own body. Like any other aspect of our health, it must be exercised and maintained by us individually.

2. Expressing sexual desire makes us feel extremely vulnerable, and the invitation to sex should never be shunned or dismissed, even if one partner is not feeling sexual. If we are not feeling sexual, it is our responsibility to convey our lack of desire to our partner with love and without hurt or shame.

3. If you are not interested in sex, offer your partner your front, not your back. When your partner is feeling sexual and you are not, don't simply roll over and go to sleep. Convey your lack of sexual desire but share your love and affection. Embrace and kiss your partner before going to sleep. As discussed earlier, touching is essential for maintaining our bond with our mate, whether we are sexual or not. We can convey much loving, healing energy with our touch and our lips without being sexual.

4. Err in the direction of sex. No one should have sex when they do not want to, but often we are just not in touch with our sexual energy. Our sexual energy may not be aroused, but it remains available to us with a little effort. It is easy to burn up a lot of our energy with our family and work responsibilities. By the time we fall into bed, it is easy for one of us to be interested in sleep more than sex. If you are the sleepyhead, consider your partner's sexual desire as an opportunity to get in touch with yours, to feel your pleasurable and life-giving sexual energy. If you make Healing Love, you will find that the vast majority of the time you will be glad you did. Especially when you are both multi-orgasmic, you can have extremely satisfying sex quickly enough that you lose little sleep. If your lack of desire is the result of disharmony in the relationship, convey your need to discuss what is bothering you or see if loving touch can smooth the rough edges of your relationship. However, if one of you is truly too exhausted to have sex or uninterested for any other reason, we encourage you to do the following:

5. Choose an alternative time for lovemaking. Whether you choose Morning Prayer or schedule time over the weekend, it is important that you plan to satisfy your sexual appetites with the same planning and forethought that you would use to satisfy your physical appetites. Agree to go to bed earlier or somehow carve out time to be intentional about your sexual intentions. In addition, even if you do not wish to "have" sex, there are various ways to "be" sexual or to satisfy the partner who is feeling sexual. We discuss these in the following section.

Being Sexual Without Doing It

In addition to the above agreements, there are ways to be sexual that will allow you to harmonize the cycles of your desire when one of you has more sexual energy than the other.

MAKING LOVE WITH MOUTH AND/OR HANDS

If one partner is not interested in having intercourse but is willing to be sexual, then he or she might be willing to participate in oral or manual sex, satisfying the other partner with mouth or hands. The person who gives oral sex receives a great deal of powerful sexual energy from his or her partner. As mentioned above, the Taoists believed that a man can absorb chi from the "three peaks" of a woman's body (her tongue, her nipples, and her vagina). Similarly, a woman can absorb a man's chi from his tongue, his nipples, and his penis. Oral and manual sex will also give you the opportunity to explore your partner's genitals in ways that are often overlooked when intercourse is the main event. This is very useful when one partner is out of commission for health or other reasons. While oral or manual sex is certainly a happy alternative for the partner who wants to be sexual, it may involve too much exertion or be "too" sexual for a partner who is tired or not interested in sex. For this reason, there is always solo cultivation in the arms of your beloved.

SOLO CULTIVATION IN THE ARMS OF YOUR BELOVED

When one partner is not interested or is too tired for the kind of energetic involvement described above or simply as another way to be intimate, the partner who is feeling sexual can self-pleasure while being held by her or his partner.

Many people are ashamed to masturbate alone, so masturbating, or solo cultivating, as the Taoists called it, in front of your partner may seem all the more shocking. In fact, it is a marvelous way to show your partner what you enjoy and to overcome the shame that many people feel about masturbating. Solo cultivation loses much of its stigma and isolation when it is brought out of the closet (or bathroom). Your partner can hold you or simply put their hands on your body. They may even choose to join in and caress you as they see how much fun you're having, but this should not be expected.

In one of the studies we cited earlier, over 70 percent of married men and women masturbate. Self-pleasuring does not take the place of marital sex but is a valuable complement. If you can have an open discussion about this natural part of human sexuality and even bring it into your bedroom, you will be able to harmonize your sexual cycles and bridge differences in desire that cause major rifts for other couples.

SOLO CULTIVATION BY YOURSELF

If you are not interested in solo cultivating in front of your partner or your partner is not interested in holding you while you cultivate, you can always get out of bed and pleasure yourself elsewhere. Remember, solo cultivation is about maintaining your sexual energy and sexual health. Just because your partner doesn't want to exercise doesn't mean you shouldn't. If your partner was not interested in going for a jog, you would still want to go. According to the Tao, each of us has yin and yang, feminine and masculine energy, and we can join these two aspects together as we make love to ourselves.

MASSAGE

If being sexual is the problem but exhaustion is not, you can exchange massages with your partner. Massage is a wonderful and important comple-ment to sex and should be included in the whole range of your loving even when you are regularly making love. As you massage your partner, try alter-nating between deeper pressure and a lighter feather touch. If your partner is too tired to exchange massages, you can offer to give him or her a massage. Often we try to get all of our needs for touch met through sex. Touching and being touched both release oxytocin and lead to a sense of well-being. If your partner does not want to touch, you can offer to do the touching. Your part-ner may even be willing to allow you to stimulate yourself on his or her body. Rubbing your genitals on your partner's buttocks, leg, or back can be highly pleasurable and can conclude a very enjoyable massage for all concerned.

TOUCH

Even if one or both of you are too tired for lovemaking of any sort or for massage, we strongly recommend that you take a few minutes or even just a few moments to touch and kiss before going to sleep. This will allow you to harmonize your energy and to reconnect after days of separation (physically or emotionally).

Touch, as you know by now, is important biochemically and energetically. When you embrace and kiss, send your partner healing love wherever you are touching. (Remember the energy that we convey with our eyes and our smile.) The release of oxytocin that occurs when you touch each other will increase your affection and your bonding with each other.

Lifelong Lovemaking

Connected as they were to the natural world, the Taoists saw our lives as divided into seasons: spring, summer, fall, and winter. But they were also pas-sionately committed to the search for longevity and even immortality. As we discussed in chapter 5, the Taoists found in the bedroom a fountain of youth that they knew to be as important in older age as it is in youth. Their beliefs have been confirmed by many recent studies, some of which we discussed in our earlier chapter. Indeed, the Taoists believed that people should make love until the day they die.

In our culture we glorify young sexuality and denigrate older sexuality. Indeed, older men who remain sexually desirous are called dirty old men. We assume that men's sexual power peaks in adolescence and then declines ever after, but this comes from a general misunderstanding of sexual power. Sexual power is not simply potency (the number of sperm) or speed to erection or the number of feet that a man can spray his ejaculate.

For the Taoists, sex was not an Olympic sport. True sexual power, they believed, is about the ability to satisfy oneself and one's partner. This ability can increase over the course of a lifetime as we understand and adjust to the physiological changes that inevitably take place. There are many things that men can do to maintain their interest in and pleasure with sex as they get older.

In our culture, older women also are assumed to lose all interest in sex, and postmenopausal women are traditionally called crones. While a woman's fertility peaks in early adulthood, her ability for sexual pleasure can expand throughout the course of her life. With the end of fertility in menopause many women actually find that they have increased sex drive as their relative testosterone level increases. There are certainly physiological changes that take place with menopause, but these can be accommodated or even postponed through hormone replacement therapy and other means, which we discuss below.

Contrary to the stereotypes, many older adults are having much more sex than is typically assumed. In a *Consumer Reports* survey of 4,246 men and women, 80 percent of married men and women over seventy remain sexually active. Fifty-eight percent have sex at least once a week.[1]

Sex certainly changes as we get older and our bodies change, but this is not a slippery slope toward sexual obsolescence. However, it is easy to worry about the loss of a sexual response that we relished in our adolescence or young adulthood. The mistake we make is in assuming that our sexual desire is the same throughout our life. We worry when our sexuality—or our partner's sexuality—changes from what we have become accustomed to.

As hormone research is making ever clearer, our sexual desire changes dramatically over the course of our lifetime, and these changes will differ greatly between the sexes and between individuals based on their hormonal profiles. What is important to remember is that each sexual stage and each

The Taoists believed that people should make love until the day they die.

80 percent of married men and women over seventy remain sexually active. 58 percent have sex at least once a week.

decade offers its own unique passionate possibilities. In fact, each new stage offers the opportunity for a more profound relationship if we are able to overcome the difficulties that occur during the tense time of transition.

The stereotypes of men wanting sex and women wanting romance are actually less true as men and women age. As men get older their testosterone level decreases and women's testosterone level (relative to their other hormones) increases. According to the language of the Tao, men become more yin, and women become more yang. As a result, men and women actually become more compatible as they age and as their hormonal differences become less extreme.[2]

Love Just Gets Better and Better

For Taoists, the goal of our love lives is ever-increasing intimacy and spiritual growth. Because Healing Love is based on the ecstatic exchange of subtle energy and not on the aerobic frenzy of pounding flesh, sexual satisfaction is not based on having a nubile body. While the frenzy is fun while it lasts and wonderful when it returns, Taoists know it is only one way of sharing love with one's partner.

According to Taoists, it takes seven years to know your partner's body, seven years to know your partner's mind, and seven years to know your partner's spirit.

According to the Taoists, it takes years to reach the heights of physical, emotional, and spiritual union. It was often said that it takes seven years to know your partner's body, seven years to know your partner's mind, and seven years to know your partner's spirit. According to the Tao, it takes twenty-one years just to get acquainted! The longer we are together the more we know each other and the better our bond can be.

This ancient insight was echoed in a university study of long-term marriages in which researchers found that, contrary to our cultural stereotypes, "old love is the best love." Robert W. Levenson, psychology professor at the University of California, Berkeley, concluded,

> *What we actually thought we would see is a kind of fatigue quality in these relationships. But that's not what we see. They're vibrant, they're alive, they're emotional, they're fun, they're sexy, they're not burned out.*[3]

According to another recent study of older adults, sexually active seniors are the happiest men and women. But to remain sexually active, you need to maintain your sexual health and learn how to respond to your body's different physiologic needs.

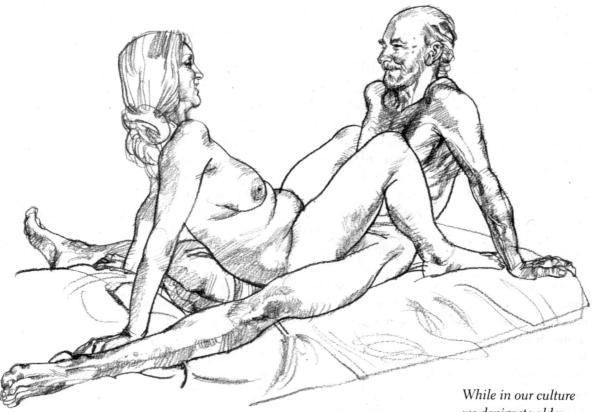

While in our culture we denigrate older sexuality, the Taoists believed that people should make love until the day they die.

Sexual Health for Older Women

BEFORE THE "PAUSE"

Significant changes in desire and sexual response frequently occur around menopause. Sex hormones begin to decline in women ten to fifteen years prior to when their periods stop, usually between the ages of forty and fifty. Usually these women have had very satisfying sexual lives and note a decrease in their sexual desire and ability to have orgasms.

In addition to the decrease in sexual hormones, this time of life can include many different stressful demands, such as young children, aging parents, career responsibilities, and so forth. Because of this, in part, the forties and early fifties are the most common age for women to become clinically depressed, which dramatically affects their sex drive. It is important at this time to consult a physician if your changing hormonal levels necessitate medical treatment. Many women who have not yet reached the menopausal stage may benefit from low-dose oral contraceptives, which will increase their estrogen level and their sexual desire.[4]

MENOPAUSE

With the gradual onset of menopause, women suffer further symptoms from the often-dramatic decrease of estrogen. Many women experience hot flashes, anxiety, insomnia, and mood swings. As if this weren't enough to affect their sex drive, many physiological changes take place in women's sexual organs. Significant thinning of the vaginal tissues occurs, leading to frequent vaginal infections and itching. Compounding the problem, this estrogen withdrawal causes reduced lubrication in the vagina.

Fortunately, many of these sexual problems can be remedied through hormone replacement therapy or alternative methods. It is worth mentioning that should you choose to do nothing, for most women the hot flashes, anxiety, insomnia, and mood swings tend to go away after the transition to menopause is complete (usually within one to two years after menstruation stops). Unfortunately, the thinning of the vaginal wall and the decrease in lubrication, which can sometimes cause pain with intercourse and more frequent infections, remain. These changes, however, can be minimized by the use of a good lubricant and by more gentle thrusting during intercourse. Topical estrogen creams can also help with vaginal irritation and dryness. As mentioned above, after women finish going through menopause, their relative testosterone level is higher and some women experience a resurgence in their desire.

After women finish going through menopause, their relative testosterone level is higher and some women experience a resurgence in their desire.

Hormone replacement therapy is an important option for many menopausal women. It has been shown to increase desire, sensitivity, and both frequency and intensity of orgasm.[5] It also alleviates the symptoms of menopause discussed above as long as the hormone therapy is continued. Unfortunately, long-term studies on the effects of hormone replacement therapy are not yet available. Though it appears safe in the great majority of women, there is still some concern about increasing the likelihood of breast cancer. Hormone replacement therapy reduces the risk of osteoporosis and fractures, but its effects on heart disease and stroke remain unclear. Studies are being done that will clarify these risks.[6] If you are interested in considering hormone replacement therapy, you should discuss your options and risk factors with your physician.

Hormone replacement therapy improves sexual enjoyment for most women. However, many women still experience a decline in their sexual desire after menopause. This is because estrogen, the hormone being replaced, is only one of the hormones that decreases during menopause. Testosterone and its cousin, DHEA, also decrease, causing a waning in sex drive. There are good studies that show that for short periods of time testosterone replacement significantly improves sex drive and overall sexual satisfaction (as well as mood) in women after menopause. Testosterone is most widely available for women in combination with estrogen in tablet form. Unfortunately, oral testosterone may not be effective in the long term and may be associated with some significant health risks.[7] Newer and safer forms of testosterone replacement therapy will be available in the near future.

For those women who choose not to take hormone replacement therapy, other supplements are available that can ease the transition to menopause. Phytoestrogens are natural estrogens that can be found in foods, most commonly soy products. Though they don't offer all the benefits of hormone replacement therapy, soy products added to your diet may alleviate some menopausal symptoms.[8] Natural progesterones in creams and oral forms also decrease the symptoms of menopause. The treatment of menopause is rapidly evolving, and newer, more effective products are increasingly available. While some people now believe that menopause will someday be managed like other hormonal imbalances, it is important to mention that women have been going through menopause for millennia and have continued to have active, satisfying sex lives.

While some people now believe that menopause will someday be managed like other hormonal imbalances, it is important to mention that women have been going through menopause for millennia and have continued to have active, satisfying sex lives.

Sexual Health for Older Men

While men do not have as dramatic a hormonal change as women, they also undergo significant hormonal changes in their forties and fifties that medical experts are starting to call "viropause." As mentioned earlier, a man's testosterone decreases over the course of his lifetime, and this decrease in male sexual hormones can cause many physiological changes, especially around middle age. For example, most men who are over fifty (and often younger) need significantly more direct genital stimulation to get and maintain an erection.

Most men who are over fifty (and often younger) need significantly more direct sexual stimulation to get and maintain an erection.

Gone are the days of spontaneous erections in the middle of algebra class. (Fortunately, also long gone are the days of algebra class.) Those awkward erections may have been embarrassing, but once this now-familiar sexual response changes, men may pine for its return.

A man's erection will also be less firm or will angle down more when he is fully erect. These changes in physical strength are no different from other changes that occur throughout his body. You would not expect to bench-press as much weight or run as fast at fifty as you were able to at twenty-five. Still, men's sense of personal power is closely attached to their penis and its performance in the bedroom. Men feel much more concerned about their penis than they do about their biceps. Therefore, it is worth following some general guidelines for maintaining your sexual health and having some useful techniques to assist you when the engine isn't exactly running like it used to.

REVVING THE ENGINE

Not only will older men require more direct genital stimulation; they will often take longer to get an erection and to get one again if they ejaculate. For this reason, we suggest you learn a trusty Taoist technique called Soft Entry. All men, not just older men, experience situational impotency, or the inability to get an erection, at various times in their life. One study showed that among men forty to seventy years old, over half had periodic impotence. Situational impotence may happen more often when men get older, and the Taoists knew it was a normal part of male sexuality. Working with nature was the Taoist secret to life, and so they developed the fail-safe Soft Entry technique, in which a man could enter with a soft or semi-erect penis and soon have a very happy and healthy hard-on. In the words of the Taoists, a man can "enter soft, exit hard."

> The Yellow Emperor: "I want to have intercourse, but my penis will not rise. I feel so embarrassed that my perspiration comes out like pearls. In my heart I crave to make love and I wish I could help with my hands. How can I help? I wish to hear the Tao."
>
> Su Nu, a famous female Taoist sex adviser: "Your Majesty's problem is a problem of all men."

Su Nu, the famous Taoist sexual adviser, first taught the Yellow Emperor to relax and try to harmonize with his partner. Taking the situation without fear or blaming oneself or one's partner is essential. A sense of humor can often help.

Fear, we now know, initiates what is called the adrenaline reflex, often called the fight-or-flight response. When we are afraid our body thinks we need to run or fight for our survival and therefore pumps blood away from our genitals to where it is needed to run or to defend ourselves. While this makes evolutionary sense — better not to have an erection when trying to run from a saber-toothed tiger — it only makes matters worse in the bedroom. So relax and know that you can actually "help with your hands," just as the Yellow Emperor had hoped. If you have a more chronic problem getting an erection, we suggest that you read the section in *The Multi-Orgasmic Man* entitled "Snake Charming: Overcoming Impotence."

Exercise 28

SOFT ENTRY

1. LUBRICATE: The woman must be fully lubricated. The man should pleasure her until her fluids are flowing heavily. You may also wish to use an artificial lubricant on the vagina and/or penis.

2. MAN ON TOP: It is generally easiest for the man to be on top so that gravity helps draw the blood into his penis and so that he has as much freedom to move as possible.

3. CIRCLE PENIS WITH THUMB AND FOREFINGER: The man should circle his thumb and forefinger around the base of his penis to form a finger ring. With his ring snugly around his penis, he can push the blood into its shaft and head. This will cause his penis to get firm enough to enter his partner.

4. ENTER AND BEGIN THRUSTING: With his finger ring still in place, he should carefully insert his penis into his partner's vagina and begin thrusting. The finger ring should remain on until he has a hard erection.

5. FOCUS ON THE PLEASURE: The man should continue focusing on the blood and sexual energy that are filling his penis and concentrate on the pleasurable sensations of intercourse.

6. PARTNER'S HELPING HANDS: His partner can stroke his testicles or push on his perineum (which will stimulate him and cause more blood to enter his penis) or play with his anus (if he likes anal stimulation). She can touch him in any other way that will add to his arousal. She can also kiss him, smile at him, or show her pleasure as he begins to move inside her. As mentioned above, there is no greater aphrodisiac for a man than the sound of his lover in pleasure.

7. ADJUST FINGER RING: Adjust the tightness of your finger ring as your penis begins to engorge. (To fill your erection the blood will need to come through your finger ring, so your grip should not be so tight that it prevents blood flow.)

8. REAPPLY IF NECESSARY: The man should reapply the finger ring if his erection wanes (although generally the warmth and softness of his partner's vagina will be enough to keep him hard).

While the Soft Entry technique will help men get an erection and avoid the adrenaline reflex, there are also a few other suggestions that can help in these anxious moments. First, you can try to focus on something erotic that arouses you. These arousing thoughts will crowd out the anxious ones.

In addition, you can focus your attention on your partner's pleasure and give her oral or manual sex. Focusing on your erection as you wait for it to rise is similar to watching the pot that never boils. Turning your attention to your partner's pleasure often works wonders, especially if she remembers to give you the genital stimulation that you increasingly need. Finally, talking to your partner about your erection concerns can often diffuse the tension and allow you to redirect your attention to other pleasures that can expand your sexual energy.

While testosterone naturally decreases each year in all men after peaking in the twenties, in some men it can decrease more dramatically, resulting in decreased desire, decreased erections, and shrinking testicles. Should you experience these symptoms, you should consult your physician. Testosterone replacement for men is now fairly simple and effective.

The popular new drug Viagra can also help men who are having erection problems. Taken one hour prior to sex, it improves blood flow to the penis and improves the ability to get and maintain an erection.

If you find that you are impotent all of the time, you should consider the possibility that you may have a physiological problem. Approximately 80 percent of the time complete impotence is the result of a medical problem, many of which can be treated. You should also consult the list of medications at the end of chapter 2, which can often interfere with erection and orgasmic ability. You can do a simple at-home test to see if you have erections in your sleep, as most men do when they are dreaming. Lick a strip of stamps and circle the base of your flaccid penis with them. If you awake the next morning and the stamps are broken, you have had a normal erection. If your stamps are unbroken, you should seek medical help from your physician.

EJACULATION AND AGING

As men age, their urge to ejaculate will generally decrease. In fact, as men age and their sexual urgency decreases they are often capable of delaying ejaculation much longer than in their youth. One of the benefits of this delayed ejaculation as men get older is that they find it easier to become multi-orgasmic. In Marion Dunn and Jan Trost's recent study, half the men had become multi-orgasmic after the age of thirty-five. These older multi-orgasmic men were all over fifty and going strong. This ability to delay ejaculation can also help older men satisfy their partner.[9]

Many men find that they no longer want to ejaculate as frequently as they did when they were younger. This, according to the Tao, is a natural and desirable change. Masters and Johnson also underscored the fact that men do not need to ejaculate every time they make love, especially men over fifty.[10] In addition, the force of a man's ejaculation will decrease and the time it takes him to get another erection (called the refractory period) will be longer as he ages.

As we mentioned in chapter 1, the famed Chinese physician Sun Ssu-miao recommended that men at forty ejaculate no more than once in ten days, men at fifty no more than once in twenty days, and men over sixty not at all. Remember, this does not prevent you from having as many *orgasms* as you wish, and when you are able to orgasm without ejaculating, you will rarely long for ejaculation. You will have all the pleasure without the sense of depletion.

Nonetheless, Sun Ssu-miao's recommendations are just guidelines. The most important measure you should use to determine how often to ejaculate is how your body feels. When you ejaculate, you should feel light and refreshed, invigorated not enervated.

Every few years, you may wish to decrease the frequency of your ejaculation, but listen to what your body tells you. And please remember, if you do ejaculate, do not beat yourself up or blame your partner. Welcome the pleasurable sensations and enjoy them. The loving exchange and joy of lovemaking is much more important than whether you do or do not ejaculate. No man should become rigid or obsessed with the frequency of his ejaculations. The goal of Healing Love is not to master the practice for its own sake but to use the practice for your overall pleasure, health, and spiritual growth.

Sexual Health for Older Couples

We have discussed a number of changes that influence your and your partner's sexual health as you get older. We have suggested a number of ways to deal with these changes to your sexuality and to keep your love life vibrant and healthy. It is also important to mention that your general physical health is also essential for your sexual health. Cardiovascular problems, for example, are the single greatest cause of impotence in men.

A healthy body and avoiding or reducing cigarettes and alcohol can dramatically improve your chances of having a long, satisfying sex life. Regular

Sex actually increases your sex hormones and your sex drive.

exercise can help prevent and treat serious diseases like high blood pressure, diabetes, and heart disease, which can seriously compromise your sex life. Exercise has also been shown to increase sex drive in both men and women.

Sex itself is an excellent form of exercise. Interestingly, it is also the best way to boost testosterone in both men and women naturally (that is, without taking additional hormones). Sex actually increases your sex hormones and your sex drive. The more you have sex, the more you want sex.

The opposite is also true, that if you go for long periods of time without sex you will have less desire for it. For this reason, you should try to be sexually active as often as possible, ideally at least once a week. If your partner is not available or is ill, you should solo cultivate. Consider it preventative medicine. As Theresa Crenshaw explains, "Both men and women who have sex often when they are younger retain the capacity to do so when they are older. However, after age sixty or so, if either one takes an extended intermission—even for a just a few months—the physical capacity for sex rapidly fades."[11] In short, as the saying goes, "Use it or lose it."

Finally, it is important to make sure that any prescription drugs that you or your partner is taking do not cause sexual problems. It is estimated that one-quarter of all impotence is caused by prescription drugs that men take for heart disease, high blood pressure, depression, and other medical conditions. These same drugs can also cause sexual problems for women, including decreasing the ability to orgasm. There are often other drugs that will not adversely affect sex drive and may even improve it. Make sure that you ask your doctor explicitly if there are any *sexual* side effects to the drugs that he or she is prescribing. A list of the most common offending drugs can be found at the end of chapter 2.

Maintaining the Charge

As we have mentioned above, the hormonal differences between men and women decrease as they get older. In the language of the Tao, as the man becomes more yin and the woman becomes more yang, the energetic polarity between them is reduced. While this can lead to you and your partner becoming increasingly compatible in bed and in your life, it can also reduce the charge or attraction between you.

According to the Tao, our attraction to our partner is partly based on the strength of this yin-yang charge. The stronger the charge, the more intense the passion. The decrease in this charge is one of the main reasons that many relationships become less exciting or arousing. It is also the reason why these same relationships may experience a rekindling of passion after one partner has been away on a business trip. Separation tends to recharge the polarity. Many couples also find that sleeping in separate beds or rooms for periods of time or permanently can increase their charge and attraction to each other.

When a man ejaculates he loses much of his yang charge, so as a man learns to control his ejaculation, couples find that they often have greater polarity. In addition, the Healing Love practice of learning to circulate and exchange sexual energy will help profoundly in maintaining the electrical charge and sexual passion in your relationship.

Finding the Way

Making Love for a Lifetime

- Be sexual (with your partner or with yourself) as often as possible, ideally at least once a week, to keep your sexual equipment and hormones primed.

- Touch each other often to keep your oxytocin and affection flowing.

- Make sure the man gets enough genital stimulation.

- Use the Soft Entry technique when needed.

- Make sure the woman has enough lubrication.

- Consider hormone replacement therapy.

- Reduce the number of times a man ejaculates.

- Maintain the sexual polarity between you.

- Avoid cigarettes, alcohol, and prescription drugs that have negative sexual side effects.

Avoid Increasing Sexual Stakes

The Taoists believed that our lovemaking could continue to improve over the course of our lifetime, and they devoted themselves to exploring the heights of sexual pleasure and intimacy. In this book we have introduced many new sexual heights, but we want to emphasize the importance of not raising the sexual stakes for you and your partner. These heights can be experienced when you and your partner are ready and willing. Try to avoid burdening yourselves with the expectation that there is some sexual goal that you must reach each time you make love.

With every new "breakthrough" in women's sexuality, from the "discovery" of women's orgasms to the G spot to the potential for women's multiple orgasms, women were expected to experience these pleasures or risk being seen as sexually inadequate. With the introduction of the possibility of multiple orgasms for men in our first book, we tried to urge men not to add to their or their partner's expectations. Knowing that sexual peaks exist allows people to climb them, but expecting yourself to climb to the top every time creates an unhelpful and unnecessary burden.

In this book, we have expanded on many of the sexual possibilities that exist for both men and women in the hope that these options will add joy and satisfaction to your love life. We hope you will explore and enjoy them in a spirit of playfulness and adventure. The Taoist techniques are called Healing Love because what is most important is focusing on healing and love. If you focus on a desire to love and heal your partner, you will certainly reach the pleasurable heights of lovemaking together.

The Arts of the Bedchamber can be cultivated over the course of a lifetime. Do not expect to learn them overnight, and do not expect every sexual encounter to be a masterpiece. Keep your excitement high and your expectations low. Try to avoid taking yourselves or your practice too seriously. Don't forget to play with each other and to keep lovemaking fun as well as profound.

The Real Secret of Sexuality

The real secret of the Tao is that there is no goal in life or in lovemaking. Life is a continually unfolding mystery, as are our relationships with one another. Multiple orgasms can indeed change the focus of lovemaking from the urgent and singular goal of achieving orgasm to the ecstatic process of intimately knowing and being known by your partner. In the end, Healing

Love is not based on the quantity of orgasms you have but on the quality of the love and healing that you experience in your relationship with your partner. Once you can have as many orgasms as you wish, you are able to realize that the orgasmic pulsations themselves are simply part of a continual process of harmonizing with your partner and with the world.

Sharing Secrets

The philosophy and practices that we have taught in this book were closely guarded secrets for many thousands of years. We have shared them because we believe that they can benefit human culture in general. Too many cultures around the world have lost their sexual wisdom, and as a result most of us are left groping in the dark for pleasure and satisfaction. According to the Tao, our sexuality is the foundation of our overall health. Any genuine healing for ourselves and for the world must begin in the bedroom, for it is through love and sex that the next generation is conceived.

We hope you will respect the power in these practices and value them no less because you did not have to study for many years with a Taoist master to learn them. If you cherish them, they will offer you and your partner great riches of joy and pleasure. We urge you to read, reread, and share them with your partner (and others you think will benefit from them). We hope that you will find in these teachings a source of Healing Love with your partner that will transform your relationship with each other and with the world.

Once you can have as many orgasms as you wish, you are able to realize that the orgasmic pulsations themselves are simply part of a continual process of harmonizing with your partner and with the world.

Any genuine healing for ourselves and for the world must begin in the bedroom, for it is through love and sex that the next generation is conceived.

INTRODUCTION

1. Alfred Kinsey was the first to report that men could experience multiple orgasms. For more on Kinsey's pioneering research see chapter 1 below or see his classic work: Alfred C. Kinsey, Wardell B. Pomeroy, and Clyde E. Martin, *Sexual Behavior in the Human Male* (Philadelphia: W. B. Saunders, 1948), pp. 158–59. William Hartman and Marilyn Fithian were the first to document male multiple orgasms in the laboratory. See Hartman and Fithian's *Any Man Can: The Multiple Orgasmic Technique for Every Loving Man* (New York: St. Martin's Press, 1984) or our *The Multi-Orgasmic Man* (San Francisco: HarperSanFrancisco, 1996) for more detail on male multiple orgasms.

CHAPTER ONE

1. According to the thirteenth edition of *Smith's General Urology*, orgasm includes "involuntary rhythmic contractions of the anal sphincter, hyperventilation [increased breathing rate], tachycardia [increased heart rate], and elevation of blood pressure." See *Smith's General Urology*, 13th ed., ed. Emil A. Tanagho and Jack W. McAninch (Norwalk, CT: Appleton and Lange, 1992), p. 710.

2. Alfred C. Kinsey, Wardell B. Pomeroy, and Clyde E. Martin, *Sexual Behavior in the Human Male* (Philadelphia: W. B. Saunders, 1948), pp. 158–59.

3. Kinsey et al., *Human Male*, pp. 158–59.

4. Herant A. Katchadourian, *Fundamentals of Human Sexuality*, 4th ed. (New York: Holt, Rinehart and Winston, 1985), p. 292.

5. William Hartman and Marilyn Fithian, *Any Man Can: The Multiple Orgasmic Technique for Every Loving Man* (New York: St. Martin's Press, 1984), p. 157; Marion Dunn and Jan Trost, "Male Multiple Orgasms: A Descriptive Study," *Archives of Sexual Behavior* 18, no. 5 (1989): 382.

6. Female ejaculation has been demonstrated in the laboratory over the past twenty years, since the publication of the landmark book that popularized its existence: *The G Spot and Other Recent Discoveries About Human Sexuality*, by Alice Kahn Ladas, Beverly Whipple, and John D. Perry (New York: Dell, 1983). The Taoists have long described a woman having three waters (the first water is lubrication, the second water is orgasm, and the third water is ejaculation). Generally ejaculation is experienced as a copious amount of fluid, although some woman do actually experience a spray of liquid.

CHAPTER TWO

1. P. Blumstein and P. Schwartz (1983), quoted in Julia R. Heiman, Ph.D., and Joseph LoPiccolo, Ph.D., *Becoming Orgasmic: A Sexual and Personal Growth Program for Women* (New York: Simon & Schuster, 1992), pp. 223–25.

2. The G spot is named after Dr. Ernst Gräfenberg, the first modern physician to describe it.

3. Some sex researchers compare the G spot to the male prostate gland, since they derive from the same embryonic tissue and both are made up of glands and ducts, swell when they are stimulated, and produce secretions. While female ejaculation is rare, the release of fluid from the urethra with orgasm is a natural part of some women's sexual response.

4. Beverly Whipple, William E. Hartman, and Marilyn A. Fithian, "Orgasm," in *Human Sexuality: An Encyclopedia*, ed. Vern L. Bullough and Bonnie Bullough (New York: Garland Publishing, 1994), p. 432.

5. William Masters and Virginia Johnson, *Human Sexual Response* (Boston: Little, Brown, 1966).

6. Beverly Whipple, Gina Ogden, and Barry R. Komisaruk, "Physiological correlates of imagery induced orgasms in women," *Archives of Sexual Behavior*, 21, no. 2 (1992): 121–133.

7. Having a glass of wine, a beer, or one drink a day has some health benefits and is unlikely to be harmful unless there is some history of alcohol abuse in yourself or your family. However, alcohol can impair sexual response, and we would not suggest using it routinely to get you in the mood.

8. Beverly Whipple, quoted in Anne Vachone, "Multiple Orgasms: Why One Orgasm is Never Enough: Cosmo's Guide to Making Orgasms Happen and Happen and Happen," *Cosmopolitan*, July 1998, p. 156.

9. Arnold Kegel was the physician who first recommended these exercises, in 1948, to strengthen the vaginal muscles and as a treatment for incontinence.

10. Carol Anderson Darling, Jay Kenneth Davidson Sr., and Donna A. Jennings, "The Female Sexual Response Revisited: Understanding the Multi-Orgasmic Experience in Women," *Archives of Sexual Behavior* 20, no. 6 (1991): 529.

11. Julia Heiman and Joseph LoPiccolo, *Becoming Orgasmic: A Sexual and Personal Growth Program for Women*, rev. ed. (New York: Prentice-Hall, 1988), p. 27.

12. Darling et al., "Female Sexual Response Revisited," p. 529.

13. Quoted in Susan Bakos, "Just When You Thought You Knew All There Was to Know About Orgasm," *Cosmopolitan*, August 1996, p. 148.

14. Alan P. Brauer and Donna J. Brauer, *The ESO Ecstasy Program: Better, Safer Sexual Intimacy and Extended Orgasmic Response* (New York: Warner Books, 1990), pp. 103–9.

15. Brauer and Brauer, *ESO Ecstasy Program*, p. 70.

16. Joy Davidson, "You Always Have Orgasms . . . Then Suddenly You Don't," *Cosmopolitan*, December 1996, 90.

17. Some IUDs release progesterone into the uterus and may have some small effect on sex drive. IUDs are available without hormonal components.

18. The IUD, though it does not increase the risk of sexually transmitted diseases, can cause a much more severe infection if you do contract one. An infection of the uterus and fallopian tubes (pelvic inflammatory disease) can cause scarring, which may compromise future fertility.

19. Linda DeVillers, as quoted in "Sexual Satisfaction Guaranteed," *Redbook*, November 1996, p. 74.

CHAPTER THREE
1. Felice Dunas, *Passion Play* (New York: Riverhead Books), p. 53.

CHAPTER FOUR
1. See Theresa Crenshaw's excellent book, *The Alchemy of Love and Lust: How Our Sex Hormones Influence Our Relationships* (New York: Simon & Schuster, 1997).

2. Crenshaw, *Alchemy of Love and Lust*, p. 96.

3. Crenshaw, *Alchemy of Love and Lust*, p. 122.

4.   Robert T. Michael, John H. Gagnon, Edward O. Laumann, and Gina Kolata, *Sex in America* (Boston: Little, Brown, 1994), pp. 158–65.

5.   P. Blumstein and P. Schwartz, quoted in *Becoming Orgasmic: A Sexual and Personal Growth Program for Women*, by Julia R. Heiman, Ph.D., and Joseph LoPiccolo, Ph.D. (New York: Simon & Schuster, 1992), pp. 223–25.

CHAPTER FIVE

1.   Susan Crain Bakos, "Just When You Thought You Knew All There Was to Know About Orgasm," *Cosmopolitan*, August 1996, p. 148.

2.   While it was not clear from the study whether the men were ejaculating each time, we assume they probably were. This study suggests that ejaculatory sex is still better than no sex. From a Taoist perspective, the sex would have been even healthier and more healing had they minimized ejaculation. *British Medical Journal*, December 20, 1997, vol. 315, no. 7123, p. 1641; "Sex and Death: Are They Related? Findings from the Caerphilly Cohort Study." George Davey Smith; Stephen Frankel; John Yarnell.

3.   Theresa L. Crenshaw, M.D., *The Alchemy of Love and Lust: How Our Sex Hormones Influence Our Relationships* (New York: Simon & Schuster, 1997), pp. 4–5.

4.   Daniel P. Reid, *The Tao of Health, Sex, and Longevity: A Modern Practical Guide to the Ancient Way* (New York: Simon & Schuster, 1989), p. 290.

CHAPTER SIX

1.   Theresa L. Crenshaw, M.D., *The Alchemy of Love and Lust: How Our Sex Hormones Influence Our Relationships* (New York: Simon & Schuster, 1997), p. 95.

CHAPTER EIGHT

1.   *Consumer Reports* survey, reported in Herant A. Katchadourian, *Fundamentals of Human Sexuality*, 4th ed. (New York: Holt, Rinehart and Winston, 1985), p. 385.

2.   For a full description of our different sexual stages and the latest hormonal research, we strongly recommend the excellent work of Theresa Crenshaw, particularly "Sexual Stages," in *Alchemy of Love and Lust*, pp. 18–52.

3.   Reported in the *Los Angeles Times*, June 4, 1995.

4.   As we have said previously, testosterone is primarily responsible for active female libido, but supplemental estrogen plays an important role in augmenting sexual interest and improving orgasmic ability.

5.   Increased desire in 90 percent of women, sensitivity in 50 percent of women, orgasm frequency in 30 percent of women, and orgasm intensity in 40 percent of women. See Maida Taylor, M.D., M.P.H., "Sex, Drugs, and Growing Old: Sexual Dysfunction in Perimenopause, Menopause, and Post-Menopause: Physiology, Psychology, and Pharmacology" (paper presented at Current Issues in Women's Health Conference, Sacramento, CA, 1999).

6.   Recent studies call into question the benefits of hormone replacement therapy for reducing heart disease, particularly in the first two years of therapy. Because the field of hormone replacement therapy is rapidly evolving, we suggest that you consult your physician for the most current information.

7.   Unfortunately, oral testosterone decreases your good cholesterol (HDL) and increases your bad cholesterol (LDL). In addition, there are no long-term studies that show that it improves sex drive after more than three months. There is also some question about its effect on breast cancer. Topical forms of testosterone, which do not affect cholesterol

levels, will soon become available. If you are interested in testosterone replacement therapy, please discuss the current available options with your physician.

8.   Phytoestrogens and natural progesterones do not increase bone density and are not as effective as hormone replacement therapy in relieving menopausal symptoms.

9.   Marion Dunn and Jan Trost, "Male Multiple Orgasms: A Descriptive Study," *Archives of Sexual Behavior* 18, no. 5 (1989): 385.

10.   Masters and Johnson, *Human Sexual Inadequacy,* quoted in Jolan Chang, *The Tao of Love and Sex: The Ancient Chinese Way of Ecstasy* (New York: Dutton, 1977), p. 21.

11.   Crenshaw, *Alchemy of Love and Lust,* p. 282.

The Healing Love practices in this book are part of a complete system of physical, emotional, and spiritual development called the Universal Tao, which is based on the practical teachings of the Taoist tradition. Following is a list of other Universal Tao books written by Mantak Chia.

Universal Tao Books

Healing Love Through the Tao: Cultivating Female Sexual Energy (with Maneewan Chia)

Taoists Secrets of Love: Cultivating Male Sexual Energy (with Michael Winn)

Taoist Ways to Transform Stress into Vitality

Awaken Healing Light of the Tao (with Maneewan Chia)

Awaken Healing Energy Through the Tao

Tao Yin

The Inner Structure of Tai Chi: Tai Chi Kung I (Juan Li)

Bone Marrow Nei Kung: Iron Shirt Chi Kung III (with Maneewan Chia)

Chi Nei Tsang: Internal Organ Chi Massage (with Maneewan Chia)

Chi Self-Massage: The Taoist Way of Rejuvenation

Fusion of the Five Elements (with Maneewan Chia)

Iron Shirt Chi Kung I: Internal Organs Exercise

To order Universal Tao books, audiocassettes, CDs, posters, or videotapes in the United States, call Universal Tao Fulfillment at 201–343–5350 or fax 201–343–8511. Outside the United States, you can write, call, fax, or e-mail the Universal Tao Center, 274 Moo 7, Laung Nua, Doi Saket, Chiang Mai 50220, Thailand. Ph. 66–53–495–596 or 66–53–865–034. Fax from Asia 66–53–495–853; fax from Europe 31–20–524–1374; fax from North America 1–212–504–8116.

E-mail: universaltao@universal-tao.com or visit the Web sites: www.multi-orgasmic.com and www.universal-tao.com.

Universal Tao Instructors and Classes

There are more than twelve hundred Universal Tao instructors through-out the world who teach classes and workshops in various practices, from

Healing Love to tai chi to chi-kung. For more information about instructors and workshops in your area, you can call toll free in the United States at 888–444–7426 or 888–841–8881. (Outside the United States but for instructors in North or South America, call 212–330–7876.) For instructors in Europe, Asia, or Australia, contact the Universal Tao Center, above. You can also find an instructor on the Web at www.taoinstructors.org..

General Sex Books

Theresa L. Crenshaw, M.D. *The Alchemy of Love and Lust: How Our Sex Hormones Influence Our Relationships.* New York: Simon & Schuster, 1997.

A truly marvelous explanation of the impact that our hormones have on our sexuality throughout the stages of our life. Dr. Crenshaw keeps the research relevant to ordinary people's lives and presents a wealth of information that every couple should know.

Paul Joannides. *The Guide to Getting It On! America's Coolest & Most Informative Book About Sex.* Waldport, OR: Goofy Foot Press, 1999.

The best general sex guide that we have found. Joannides offers over six hundred pages of detailed and humorous sex advice. As fun to read as it is useful, Joannides's book tells you how to do things that you may never have heard of with parts of your body you may not have known you had.

Alan P. Brauer, M.D., and Donna J. Brauer. *The ESO Ecstasy Program: Better, Safer Sexual Intimacy and Extended Orgasmic Response.* New York: Warner Books, 1990.

The Brauers are two of the leading sex researchers who have studied extending orgasmic pleasure. Their program and their 1982 best-seller, *ESO,* are excellent guides for intensifying pleasure.

Women's Sex Books

Mantak and Maneewan Chia. *Healing Love Through the Tao: Cultivating Female Sexual Energy.* Huntington, NY: Healing Tao Books, 1991.

A more advanced guide to working with female sexual energy that teaches women how to enhance their sexuality and decrease the pain and depletion that often accompany menstruation.

Julia R. Heiman, Ph.D., and Joseph LoPiccolo, Ph.D. *Becoming Orgasmic: A Sexual and Personal Growth Program for Women.* New York: Simon & Schuster, 1992.

The best program we have found for helping women who have never had an orgasm.

Alice Kahn Ladas, Beverly Whipple, and John D. Perry. *The G Spot and Other Recent Discoveries About Human Sexuality.* New York: Dell, 1983.

A classic. Even after almost two decades this book still has a great deal of valuable advice about women's sexuality.

Joani Blank. *The Good Vibrations Guide: The Complete Guide to Vibrators.* Burlingame, CA: Down There Press, 1989.

If you need a helping hand.

Men's Sex Books

Mantak Chia and Douglas Abrams. *The Multi-Orgasmic Man: Sexual Secrets Every Man Should Know.* San Francisco: HarperSanFrancisco, 1996.

The original book for men who want to be multi-orgasmic and their partners who want to help them. Please see the description and reader comments on page 205.

Mantak Chia and Michael Winn. *Taoist Secrets of Love: Cultivating Male Sexual Energy.* New York: Aurora Press, 1984.

A more advanced guide to working with male sexual energy that teaches men to develop greater sexual and personal mastery.

Bernie Zilbergeld, Ph.D. *The New Male Sexuality.* New York: Bantam Books, 1992.

A valuable book for understanding male sexual psychology as well as biology.

Taoist Sex Books

Felice Dunas. *Passion Play: Ancient Secrets for a Lifetime of Health and Happiness Through Sensational Sex.* New York: Riverhead Books, 1997.

An excellent explanation of Taoist sexuality and its relationship to the overall health of the body by a well-known acupuncturist.

Daniel P. Reid. *The Tao of Health, Sex, and Longevity: A Modern Practical Guide to the Ancient Way.* New York: Simon & Schuster, 1989.

Sex is just one small piece of this enormously helpful guide to Taoist practices of health and longevity.

Joseph Kramer. *Fire on the Mountain: An Intimate Guide to Male Genital Massage.* Videocassette. EroSpirit Research, P.O. Box 3893, Oakland, CA 94609.

A superb guide to penis massage, the video is made for gay couples but is just as useful for heterosexual couples.

Erotica

Anaïs Nin. *Delta of Venus: Erotica.* New York: Bantam Books, 1978.
Still the classic book of women's erotica. A literary feast for the imagination.

Lonnie Barbach, Ph.D., ed. *Erotic Interludes: Tales Told by Women.* New York: Plume, 1995.
Great women-focused contemporary erotica.

Lonnie Barbach, Ph.D., ed. *The Erotic Edge: 22 Erotic Stories for Couples.* New York: Penguin Books, 1996.
Erotic stories by men and women that are great to share with your partner.

Susie Bright, ed. *The Herotica Series: Collections of Women's Erotic Fiction.* New York: Penguin, 1994–.
Excellent collections by and for straight, lesbian, and bisexual women.

Catalogs and Internet Sites (for vibrators and more)

Good Vibrations: www.goodvibes.com
    800-289-8423

Adam & Eve: www.aeonline.com
    800-274-0333

Eve's Garden: www.evesgarden.com

Stockroom: www.stockroom.com

Xandria Collection: www.xandria.com
    800-242-2823

The Multi-Orgasmic Man:
Sexual Secrets Every Man Should Know

By Mantak Chia and Douglas Abrams

Reader comments for *The Multi-Orgasmic Man:*

"No man should have sex until he reads this book!!! This book absolutely changed my life. The info that I applied in this book was surprisingly easy to learn and use. I believe that if you want to be good at something you have to study it and this was a great place to start concerning my sexuality. My only regret is that I wasn't exposed to this book a long time ago!"

—A reader from Rolla, Missouri

"If you don't buy this book you're making a mistake. This is undoubtedly one of the most surprising things I have ever learned. This really works. Males can have multiple orgasms. This is one book that I will be glad I have read for the rest of my life (not to mention the appreciation my girlfriend has for this book). If you do not buy this book, you are making a mistake. The techniques laid out in this book are something every man should know!"

—A reader from San Diego, California

"The technique works! This is the first book like this I have ever read—and it may be the last. Although I am generally skeptical of this sort of 'self-help' book, this one is everything it claims to be. I am absolutely amazed that a technique such as the one this book describes could be so easily workable. To say the least, my wife has enjoyed the book every bit as much as I have, and she hasn't even read it yet!"   —A reader from Salt Lake City, Utah

"A must-read for men (and women) of all ages. I read this book before encouraging my husband to read it. The chapter for women is an added blessing. I plan on allowing my teenage son to read it, possibly for the bene-fit of my someday future daughter-in-law."   —A reader from Massachusetts

"You'll be begging for more. This book expands the realm of possibility. . . . Run, don't walk . . . buy this book for yourself and then make your significant other read it as well."   —A reader from San Francisco, California

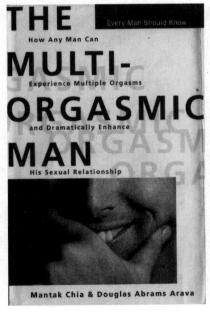